A Journey in the Fog of Depression: A Military Spouse's Experience

Kind regards,

By,
Sharon T. Kruder
and
Captain Todd G. Kruder, USN

A Journey in the Fog of Depression:
A Military Spouse's Experience

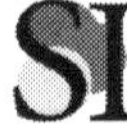

Distributed by Seurat Innovations, LLC
www.seuratinnovations.com

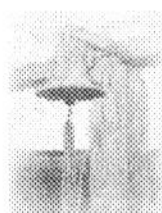

A Companion Company of Lucius Seneca Wellness Group, Inc.
www.LuciusSenecaWG.org

Sharon T. Kruder
and
Captain Todd G. Kruder, USN

The views presented herein are those solely of the author(s) and do not necessarily represent the views of DoD or its Components.

Seurat Innovations, LLC, Prince Frederick, Maryland

Please note this publication is based on personal experience. Although the author(s) and publisher(s) have made every reasonable attempt to achieve complete accuracy of the content in this publication, they assume no responsibility for errors or omissions.

You should use the information contained in this book as you see fit, and at your own risk. Your particular situation may not be exactly suited to the life experiences illustrated here; in fact, it is likely that they will not be the same, and you should adjust your use of the information accordingly.

Any trademarks, service marks, product names or named features is assumed to be the property of their respective owners, and are used only for reference. There is no implied endorsement if we use one of these terms.

Nothing in this book is intended to replace common sense, legal, medical or other professional help, and is meant solely to inform the reader.

Please look for the release of future publications, like this one, from Seurat Innovations, LLC, a social enterprise, **www.SeuratInnovations.com**

Seurat Innovations is a proud, for profit, Companion Company of Lucius Seneca Wellness Group Inc., a Non-Profit, Social Enterprise.
www.LuciusSenecaWG.org

Dedication

Dedicated to the spouses of our Military active duty and veterans. May they find solace in these writings and hope to continue their own personal journey through the fog of depression.

Foreword

The following content was written solely by Sharon T. Kruder a military spouse of over 25 years. Mrs. Kruder dutifully served alongside her husband, a military Navy Officer, through numerous deployments and travel. CAPT and Mrs. Kruder are parents of five children, all born whilst CAPT Kruder served on active duty.

Todd and I have been through a lot together these past twenty-six years. Our marriage has been tested. Our life constantly changing. Today as I write this our marriage is stronger. Although, just like our life, it too is a work in progress.

I hope others who read this book, who may have a significant other, who may be suffering from depression, will know this; you are NOT alone. There are others who are experiencing the difficulties associated with this illness.

I've been asked, "Why in the world would you do this? Why risk the embarrassment?" I simply reply, "It's important to both my husband and I to break the stigma associated with depression. You're no less of a person for seeking help. We must get to a point within our culture that we accept Behavioral Health therapist visits as much as we accept going to the doctor or the dentist.

Todd suffered for years with his illness. He stopped his therapy several times due to societal stigma as well as some unique military influences. Todd struggled with the knowledge that his flight pay and flight status would be affected by continued treatment. Not only did I have to battle the societal stigmas of depression, I had to contend with these unique military influences as well. I tried to convince him that money wasn't everything and he was no less of a man for admitting he suffered from depression. That he wasn't less physically qualified despite what the Navy was telling him.

I would be lying if I said there were not times when I felt helpless. How could I, a military spouse, explain to my husband after twenty plus years of service he wasn't qualified? How could I explain to him that even though he met all his flight gates he would lose his flight pay?

This brings me to other questions I have been asked, "Why did you stay? Why didn't you leave him?" My answer is simple, my marriage vows are VERY important to me. You vow in good times and in bad. Sometimes you need to work through the bad to get to the good.

The questions above is normally preceded by, "Why didn't you get him help sooner?" Sounds like it should be an easy answer. The fact is, yes, I saw Todd changing. Something changed while he was on deployment in Iraq. I noticed when Todd returned I saw he was withdrawing himself more and more. I figured this was just an adjustment phase. Similar to the many times he returned from a deployment, we adjusted. I discovered early on I could not force him to get help if he didn't want it or felt he needed it.

Todd did not want help. He could not admit to himself that he was having problems. When he finally did seek help he discovered the consequences in the military and pulled himself away from therapy.

Severe depression has a dramatic effect on our ability to think clearly and logically. Depression influences our ability to realize that suicide is not a reasonable solution to our problems. Be relentless and be persistent. Don't stop. Listen and support your spouse, wherever, and whenever it is possible.

Know that there is ALWAYS hope, you just have to find it.

Authors Note

The places, events, and people mentioned in this book are based on Sharon's and my best recollection of them, and to the best of our memories ability.

Introduction

Todd often phrased his illness as "My Depression" or "I have depression." These two phrases, although simplistic in form, connotes an ownership, a right, a sole proprietorship on the illness. Todd is quick to point out, "NOTHING and I MEAN NOTHING could be further from the truth."

Todd commented, "The illness was and still is experienced by my wife, our family, our friends, and my co-workers. Depression is unlike a cancer. It doesn't just affect you. It's not some microcosm cell dividing itself uncontrollably within your own body. No, depression effects who we are as a person. It slowly, methodically, and sometimes tragically effects our way of thinking. Our ability to rationalize thought. Because of this, depression impacts all of those who we come into contact with. Like a sneeze blown into the air by someone who suffers from a cold. It spreads."

Todd continued, "Unable to reason, unable to see this impact depression was having I continued on my journey through the fog. Believing I was the only crew member on this voyage. Every time I allowed my depression to take control of my emotions it was another slash of a scabbard across the skin of my wife and my children. In nearly the truest form of the word I created an emotional gash on their bodies. Only the swipe of my scabbard left no visual signs of bleeding or external wound to be healed. My scabbard of depression cut them emotionally, it affected who they are and how they perceive not only me, but how they perceive others in the same roll as husband and father."

In Todd's second book, *Mending the SEAM*, he describes how our experiences, life's waypoints, or Seurat Dots, could be transformed and interpreted in the same way a cardiologist interprets the results of an angioplasty procedure. Through the *SEAM* method Todd created a virtual emotional vein. By reasoning on our experiences or Seurat Dots, he depicts them in a time and space domain. "We can give our Seurat Dots depth, length, and color. We can visualize the points of constriction, in the same way a cardiologist views a constricted human vein or artery only I refer to this collection of seemingly disparate experiences as our Lucius Emotional Vein."

The Seurat Experience Dots that follow describe Sharon's own very personal experiences. Todd comments, "Someone once told me it was very courageous, to write my first book. I replied, 'Courageous, NO. It took me over five years to get help and stay with it. That's not courage to me. I will say if there is anyone on this journey how exemplifies courage it is Sharon. She's the hero in this story. She stayed with me. She saved me."

Section One
Getting to Know the Military Spouse

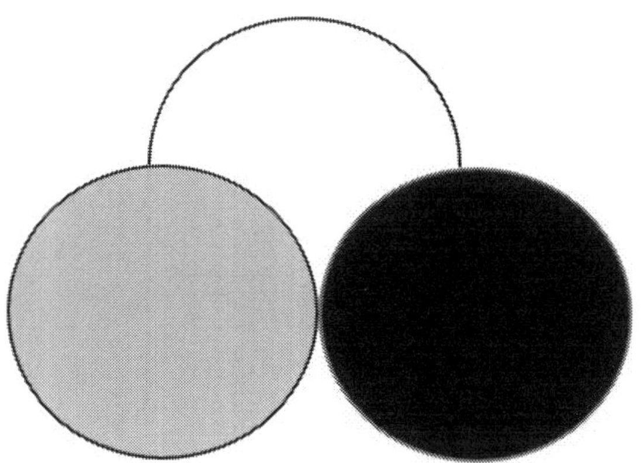

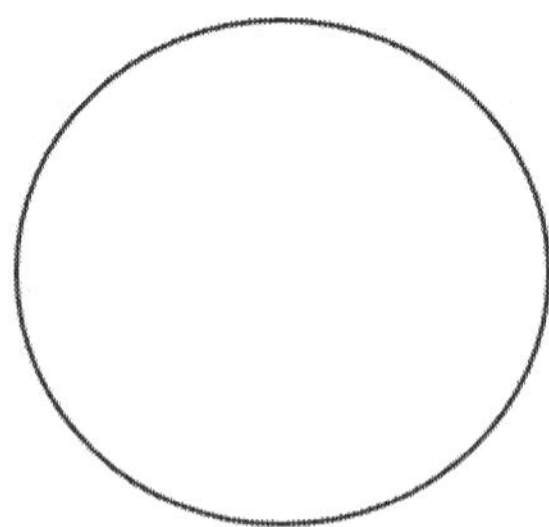

Seurat Dot One
The Origin.

This particular dot sets the *origin* of our timeline. The reference point by which all other Seurat Dots will be referenced.

Sharon is the youngest of five children and the fourth daughter. She grew up within a household of modest means in a fairly typical white collar urban setting.

Her childhood home was located on the south side of Chicago just along the city limits of Evergreen Park, literally down the street from her childhood home. Todd often commented, "It was interesting that as you drove down the street, it widened to a width more suitable for a 20th century automobile. That's when you knew you were no longer in Chicago."

Sharon's childhood neighborhood consisted of similarly constructed bungalow type homes, each distinguished by a different color of brick. A typical floor plan consisted of three bedrooms, one bath, a living room, a kitchen, and a basement. The passing of Sharon's grandmother left her grandfather in need of more care. The family decided that it was in the grandfather's best interest if he lived with them. Within six months of her grandfather's arrival an addition was added to the back of the home. The addition created two rooms and a second bath.

Sharon's father worked as a pension specialist by day, and a liquor clerk by night. The best way to describe Sharon's father is by saying he is extremely bright, quiet, hardworking, and a religious man.

Sharon's mother passed away about ten years ago after a lengthy struggle with cancer. Her mother worked in a cafeteria at the local Catholic High School. Sharon's mother could be described as, loving, kind, hardworking, and religious.

Sharon was born in Chicago like her many siblings. She lived in the same home her entire life. Just like her sisters and brother, she was raised a Roman Catholic. She attended grammar school at Saint John Fisher just like her sisters and brother. Sharon went on to attend Mother McCauley High School.

Sharon's father was a man of routine. Monday through Friday he would wake by 6:00 in the morning. Shave, shower, dress, eat a poached egg and toast all the while listening to WGN radio and Wally Philips. He would put on his overcoat (depending on the season), reach for his brief case, and walk to the local bus stop just the other side of 103rd street.

From the bus stop he would pick up the "L" or the Chicago elevated train into the heart of downtown Chicago where he faithfully performed his duties as a Pension Specialist.

Sharon's dad would do the same route just in reverse to arrive back at the house at 6:00 in the evening. Before dinner her dad or mother would have themselves a cocktail typically a Martini or Manhattan. On the days he worked the Liquor counter at Monaco, a local pharmacy on the corner of 103rd and Kedzie, he would stop home for a bite to eat and head back out once again to work his four hour shift.

Sharon's mother was by all impressions a "typical home maker". She did the laundry, the cooking, the cleaning, the grocery shopping, and of course took care of the children. As the children grew and began to go their separate ways she began to work at the local catholic boy's high school called Brother Rice. There she worked as a cafeteria employee serving lunch to the students. When she worked at the High School she would leave the house around 7:30 in the morning and return back by 2:30 in the afternoon in time to watch her favorite soap, General Hospital, catch up on the news by reading the papers, clean the house a bit, and finally prepare dinner for the evening.

Tragically Sharon's parents first born child, John, died of pneumonia only months after being born. Sharon was the youngest in a family that spanned 10 years between the oldest and herself. The oldest child was a daughter, followed by their only son, then two more daughters, and last but of course not least, Sharon.

Seurat Dot Two
Grammar School Torment

Similar to Todd's grammar school experience, Sharon attended a parochial grammar school where about sixty students were split amongst two classrooms. For the most part, over the course of eight years, these same sixty students would intermix between classrooms. This intermixing of nearly the same students over eight years created tight bonds and a fine tuned awareness of each other's strengths and weaknesses.

As was the norm for their generation, Sharon's parents maintained busy lifestyles that didn't necessarily involve direct contact with the children. Sharon grew up with little parental involvement when it came to homework and extracurricular activities such as sports. Although these activities were never frowned upon by her parents, she was often left to find her own means of transportation. Needless to say this posed a significant challenge and did nothing in the way of advocating her involvement.

With little assistance for extracurricular activities and in a time when calories were only something you learned about if you took chemistry, she began to put on weight.

There is no worse situation for a young child struggling with weight issues to be in then the dreaded Physical Education (PE) class. "PE represented the one time in the day that my lack of physical ability would be placed on display."

"In the fourth grade I had a PE teacher who was into gymnastics so much so that PE basically was gymnastics event. One event in particular I didn't like was the 'vaulting buck'. One PE period we were instructed to vault over the buck and land on your feet on the opposite side. I made my run at the vault, hitting it with weight of my two feet, and instead of propelling myself over to the other side I ended up straddling the buck. Suffice it to say this lack of gymnastics ability and total embarrassment on my part was comedic relief for those in my PE class that day."

"In another experience related to my weight, I recall one winter when we had to eat our lunches in the classroom. Before school I would pull together my lunch and place it in a typical brown paper bag. This one morning in particular we didn't have much in the house so I grabbed a can of diet root beer and placed it in my lunch. During lunch I reached into the brown paper bag and pulled out the can of pop and placed it on my desk. A couple of boys in my class sitting nearby said in a sarcastic and insincere way, 'You trying to watch what you're eating?' The other said, 'What? You trying to lose weight?' I never brought another diet soda to school again."

Seurat Dot Three
"Bennied"

Sharon attended an all-girls high school which just so happened to be conveniently located about 200 yards away from where Todd was going to school.

Jokes were played on the new freshmen. The term used at the time was, "bennied" stemming from the root word "benny" a slang term associated with being a freshman.

The pranks ranged from simple jokes, like telling someone to go take the elevator, or head to the pool, etc. Some pranks even got physical. In today's lingo the term bennied is equivalent to bullying.

A freshman, Sharon was walking down the school hallway with her books held in her hands. When from behind a group of upper classmen reached around underneath her elbow and with a swift swipe pushed her books from her grasp, spilling the contents onto the busy hallway floor.

The action was greeted with the familiar snicker and loud laughter from students passing by. Embarrassed, yes. Upset, yes. Mad, yes. All these emotions and more flowed through her body as she knelt down to the floor to retrieve her belongings.

So why was this moment so memorable for Sharon? Sharon's response, "Oh, it wasn't that I was bennied. Other girls had the same thing done to them. No. It was because my older sister and her friends, seniors, stopped, and helped me pick up my books."

This experience was important. This experience was one of "kindness." Seldom do we take the time to reflect on what was good in our life.

Section Two
How They Met

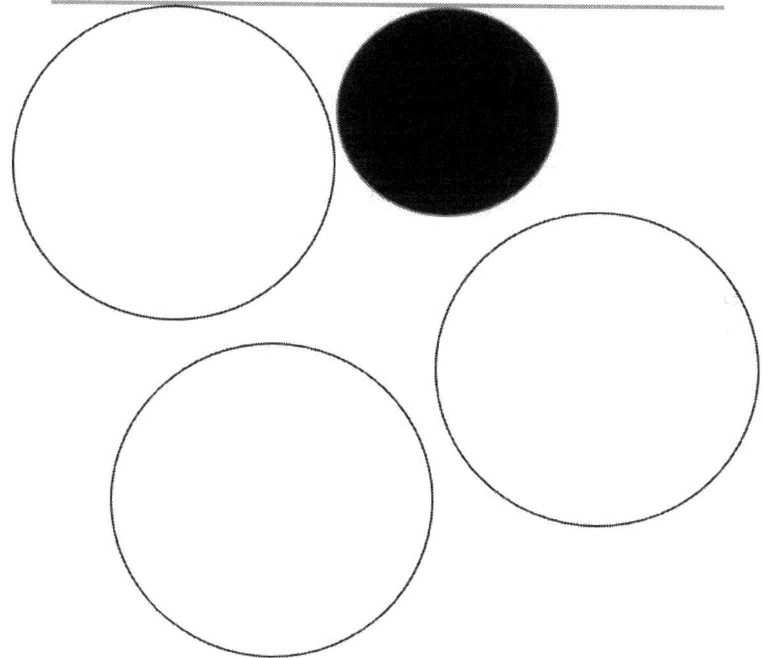

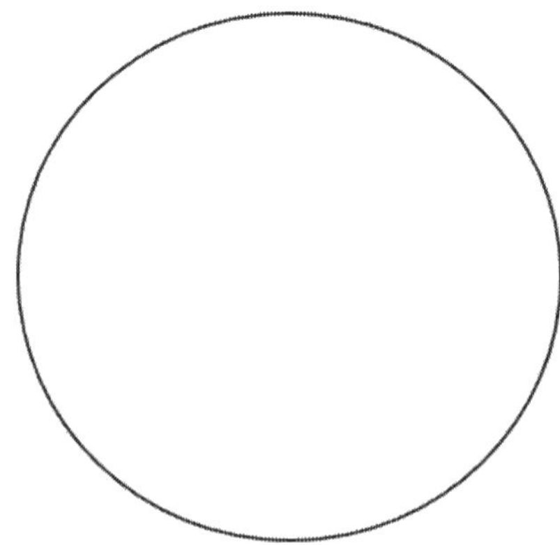

Seurat Dot Four
Favorite Root Beer

Sharon's father worked part time at a local pharmacy and convenience store called Monaco named after its owner. The weekday employees were older women while the night and weekend crew were mostly High School students.

The Liquor clerk had the undocumented responsibility of supervising the stock boys. The register clerk duties ranged from pharmacy, cosmetology, front register, and the "office" duties. "Office" had the responsibility of hourly register pickups, coverage for others while they took their breaks, and the nightly responsibility of balancing the drawers.

Working at Monaco was a legacy of sorts in Sharon's family. Her father worked there, her brother and one older sister did not get their start at Monaco. Monaco was a stepping stone, only a few hundred yards away from the house. It was an easy walk, no car required.

Of course there was the work experience and the money. Yeah, the money. Sharon started at $2.85 an hour. By the time she left the store, four years later, she was making $3.50 an hour. Sharon quickly gained the trust of the managing supervisor and within a year she was entrusted with the "keys" to the office. Incredibly, she accomplished this achievement as a junior in high school and for not much more than the starting salary of $2.85 an hour. Needless to say, Sharon is a whiz with numbers and always has been. She can calculate and remember financial numbers like nobody's business.

It just so happened a student in one of Todd's high school history class worked at Monaco. He commented one day to Todd that Monaco was looking to hire another stock boy. Todd was a junior and needed cash to help pay for gas. He saw this as just the right opportunity.

Todd started several days later. He worked about three days under the supervision of the other stock boys. He quickly learned the ropes and became familiar with the pharmacist, liquor clerks, and cashiers who worked in the front of the store.

The storeroom located just behind the pharmacy served also as a makeshift break room. It was a small five by four foot space kept clear of delivery boxes, enough space to accommodate two metal folding chairs against the wall. While on break, it was common practice for the night crew cashiers to finish homework or peruse a magazine from the store. The stock boys typically hung out with the liquor clerks. There were primarily three liquor clerks, Sharon's father was one of them. Todd had no idea he was Sharon's father, it wasn't until later that Todd learned this fact.

Sharon headed back to the break room while Todd was sweeping the storeroom floors. Todd pushed the broom across the concrete floors passing by Sharon by several times. She looked up at Todd, peering over her glasses and math book. She smiled and said to Todd, "I think you missed a spot." This was Todd's first glimpse into Sharon's sarcastic and often frustrating sense of humor. Todd stopped sweeping and said, "Thanks for the help." Sharon and Todd continued the banter for several minutes and began to laugh at each other's remarks. This began what would be a series of friendly and frequent conversations between the two of them.

Sharon picked up her soda, it was a brand of root beer. Todd asked her, "So, you like root beer?" Sharon replied, "Oh yea. But only certain kinds." Todd was intrigued be her reply, "So what kinds do you like?" Sharon immediately mentioned several of her favorite brands. They also so happened to be Todd's as well. They spent the greater portion of Sharon's break talking about root beer and shared in their disdain for one particular brand on the market at the time. Little did Sharon and Todd realize, a simple discussion about root beer would be the catalyst for a future together.

Over the weeks that followed they talked more, and more. Their conversations became personal in nature. They began to inquire into each other's family and their past.

In time Sharon began to have feelings she wanted to see more of Todd. She wanted to see him outside of Monaco. These feelings Sharon had become more prominent as senior prom for the older girls working the night shift grew closer. Sharon recalled one evening the girls talking to one another about who they might take to prom. A couple of the senior's commented, "I think I may ask Todd." Sharon realized then that Todd meant more to her than just someone to share root beer stories with. When Sharon heard this conversation she thought to herself, "I don't want to lose Todd to those girls. If he goes out with one of them I'll probably never get the chance to go out with him myself."

As the evening shift drew to a close, another stock boy who attended the same high school as Todd approached Sharon, "Hey Sharon, I'm not trying to play match maker, but Todd gave me a note to give to you." As he extended his hand toward Sharon, she could see that he was quite uncomfortable. Sharon took the piece of folded paper from his hand and said, "What is this?" He looked at Sharon and replied, "Its Todd's phone number. He wanted you to give him a call tonight. You do whatever you want." Sharon looked on the piece of paper. At first she was excited. Then she began to think, "What if this is a prank? Why would he ever want me to call him?" Variations on those thoughts continued to run through Sharon's head as she prepared to go home for the evening.

It was now 10:15 in the evening and Sharon's mother was preparing to take her to her sisters to baby sit that night. Sharon said nothing about the phone number to her mother during the ten minute drive. As her mother drove, Sharon simply starred out the car window, not talking much, still contemplating what she should do.

Now dropped off at her sister's house for the evening. Sharon's brother in law greeted Sharon at the door. Sharon's brother in law was a down to earth Italian who wouldn't hold back his opinion, an opinion that Sharon very much respected but perhaps not in this particular instance.

Her brother in law asked how she was and Sharon said, "I need to ask you your opinion about something that happened at work tonight." Her brother in law replied, "Sure. What is it?" Sharon began to recap the evening events and asked, "So, should I call him?" Her brother in law didn't hesitate to share his opinion on the matter, "It's not appropriate for you to call a guy. He should be calling you." Sharon replied, "How's he going to call me when I'm not even at home. I'm here for the evening." Sharon thought to herself, "I want him to say 'Yea that makes sense, give him a call." Since he wasn't agreeing with her Sharon spent some time still trying to decide what to do. To make matters even more complex it was now coming on 11:00 in the evening. "What if it's too late to call him? Will I wake his parents?"

Alone in the house, Sharon had to decide what she was going to do. Sharon sat in a kitchen chair near the corded phone that hung on the wall, debating what to do. Sharon mustered up the courage and dialed the number that was on the piece of now crinkled up paper. Sharon took her pointing finger and inserted it into the plastic rotary dial, her body was a bundle of nerves as she watched the dial return to zero after each number.

The phone rings once and a voice on the other end says, "Hello?" Sharon asked to speak with Todd, not knowing at the time it was he who answered the phone. Unbeknownst to Sharon, Todd had been sitting in the darken hallway at his house, his back up against the wall, anxiously waiting for her call. "I'm sorry for calling so late but he said it would be ok if I did." Todd replied, "Its fine its fine. I'm glad you called."

Sharon and Todd talked for a good hour. With it now past midnight Todd ask Sharon, "How would you feel about going to the spring dance with me?" Sharon replied, "That would be great." Sharon thought to herself, "I'm going to get to go to my first dance."

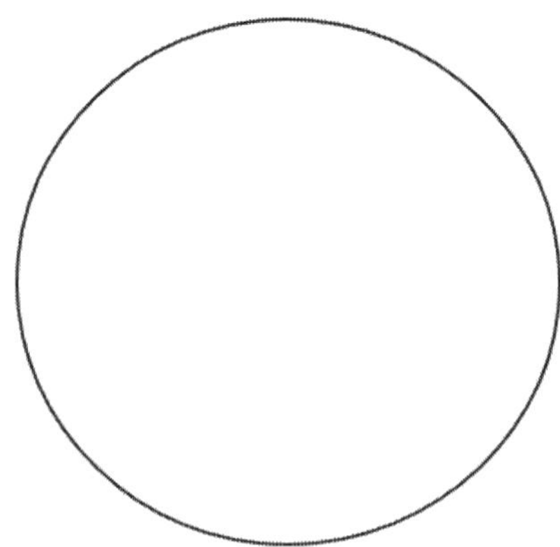

Seurat Dot Five
First Kiss

Sharon and Todd went to the spring dance during their junior year. Neither of them danced, although Sharon would have gone out on the dance floor if Todd asked.

They sat at a round table off to the side of the gym's basketball court and talked; although it was hard to hear because of the loud music playing in the background. When a slow dance was played, they would look at each other, and with agreeing eyes get up from the table and head out onto the gymnasium floor.

As the dance continued on Sharon thought to herself, "I can't believe the dance is almost over and he hasn't even tried to kiss me." Sharon began to worry, "Maybe he wasn't interested in me anymore? Maybe he just wanted a date to the dance and that was it?"

The evening came to an end and it was time to take Sharon home. Todd drove Sharon back to her home, he parked the car in front of the house, and walked Sharon to the front door. The two talked briefly, Todd leaned into Sharon, and nervously kissed Sharon good night. Sharon recalls, "When we kissed it was exhilarating and uplifting. It was simply fantastic."

Seurat Dot Six
Water Slide

Sharon and Todd had been dating for over a year. It was the summer before the start of college. Todd and Sharon would frequently double date with his older brother and his girlfriend.

It was a hot and humid Chicago summer day when one late afternoon they all decided to go to a water slide park which recently opened not far from where Todd lived. Sharon and Todd had never been to a water slide park before and were excited to go.

The water slide park was simply laid out featuring a tall wavy side-by-side slide that had a couple of bends in the middle and ended in a pool at the bottom.

The park was crowded clambering with children and adults of all ages. Although it was busy, Sharon and Todd managed to take a couple of trips down the slide without having to wait very long. Sharon, Todd, his brother, and his girlfriend thought it would be fun if they went down the slide all together.

The group of them headed up the metal stairway toward the platform at the top of the slide. A "life guard" or "monitor" sat in a folding chair where they served one primary function, to meter the flow of bodies going down the slide. Todd's brother's girlfriend sat on the slide first, followed by his brother, then Sharon, and finally Todd. They interlocked their legs and began to speed down the slippery slide. Due to the speed at which they were accelerating their legs became undone, no longer interlocked with one another. Only feet away from the bottom of the slide, their bodies were propelled into the awaiting water of the pool. Somehow Todd's brother and girlfriend made it safely into the pool, immediately standing up once their feet hit the bottom. Sharon was not so lucky. Todd's legs were thrown up into the air as he excited the slide. His legs now hanging over Sharon's shoulders with the kinetic energy of his body yet absorbed by the water.

With the force of Todd's body now acting like an anvil on Sharon's back, Sharon's body is compressed between the bottom of the pool and the weight of Todd. As soon as he could, Todd sprang to his feet, standing in the pool just behind Sharon and pulled her up by her shoulders. Sharon, now standing in the pool tried to breath but couldn't. Never before did Sharon experience what it felt like to have the "wind knocked out of you".

Sharon's face was panic-stricken; she tried desperately to catch her breath. Todd's older brother and his girlfriend rushed to Sharon's side as well. A mother of some children nearby came up to them suggesting to Sharon, "I think she should be taken to the hospital." Hearing this, Sharon refused.

They took Sharon back to the car and decided to drive back to Todd's house. Sharon was in an inordinate amount of pain, still shacking as they carried her back to the family room of the house. They placed her on her back on a couch. Sharon was in tears, wincing in pain. Todd's mother walks into the family room and see's Sharon on the couch, "What happened?" Todd replies, telling his mother about the accident. "Oh you poor thing. You need to go to the hospital. You need to go right now." Sharon wasn't going to have that as an option. She didn't want anything to do with a hospital. By now Todd knew her well enough to know that she could be very stubborn. "She could be like a mule if she wanted to be." Todd looked at her, "Sharon, you need to go to the hospital. We have to get you looked at. This isn't anything to play with. We need to go now." Sharon knew in her mind what the right thing to do was. She reluctantly agreed saying, "Ok. Ok."

They arrived at the emergency room and were joined by Sharon's mother and father. The emergency room staff immediately took Sharon back to the triage area and laid her down on a gurney. Sharon's mother stayed with her while Sharon's father and Todd remained in the waiting area.

After about two hours Sharon's mother walks out into the waiting area where she tells Todd, "The doctors want her to stay a few nights. She fractured the lower vertebrae in her back. They don't want her to go home. Of course you know Sharon. She doesn't want to stay. Maybe she'll listen to you." Todd nodded his head and followed Sharon's mother close behind up to a hospital room. They had already given Sharon something for the pain, she remained adamant she wasn't staying at the hospital, she was going home.

Sharon's mother was right. Todd managed to convince her to stay in the hospital. It was now about 2:00 in the morning. The nursing staff directed Todd to leave. Before he left he apologized once again to Sharon. Sharon looked back at Todd and replied, "It's not your fault. It was an accident. You couldn't have done anything."

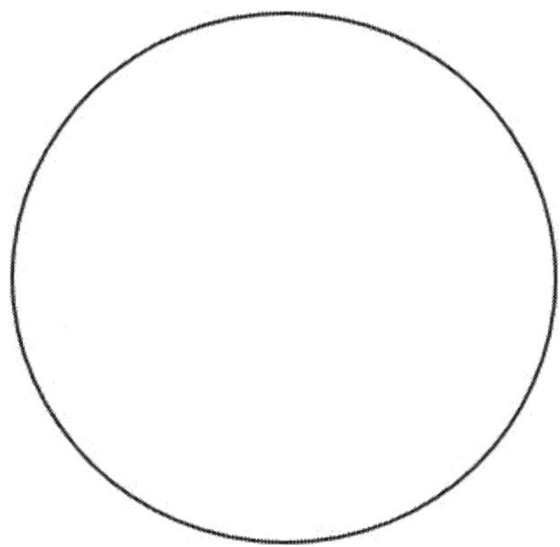

Seurat Dot Seven
Wedding Rings

Three years had passed since their first dance on the high school gym floor. As time went on, Sharon and Todd began to discuss what type of future they would have together. Todd knew that Sharon wanted an even number of children. The rationale was quite humorous. Sharon had frequented a number of amusement parks as a child and she knew what it was like to be the "odd" person out. You see, Sharon grew up in a family of seven. The amusement car rides were tailored for even numbers. Sharon always wanted an even number so that no one would ever have to sit next to a stranger; it was simple amusement park math.

Todd and Sharon were walking out of the local grocery store one summer evening. As they were walking they started to discuss Todd's future in the military and what impact it would have their future together. Todd asked, "Are you sure you're ok with me being in the military?" Sharon replied, "What do you mean?" Todd stopped and looked at Sharon, ""I mean, what about your career? Your life?" Todd was shocked by how quickly and authoritatively Sharon responded, "I know I might be putting my career aspirations on hold, but I'm ok with that. I want to be with you." Todd was simply stunned to discover that my love for him was more important than my own career. This discussion was a pivotal moment in their lives.

Following with their practical, methodical, and calculating personalities Sharon and Todd discussed at length how long the engagement would be and when they would get married. They decided on a December wedding with a two year engagement.

Their attention turned toward an engagement ring. Sharon, worked at Monaco and had little in the way of disposable income. Todd was on a Navy college scholarship with little money of his own, certainly not enough to purchase a high end ring. They knew what they could afford and going to an independent jeweler was out of the question. So they turned to retail store called *Service Merchandise*, a cutting edge store for its time. Upon entering the store the customer reached for a small clipboard that had a pencil and a sheet of paper attached. The store itself was setup like an Ikea, merchandise was displayed along the walls and along the aisles. As a customer approached a piece of merchandise they wanted to purchase, they would write a unique identification number and the desired quantity on the piece of paper attached to the clip board. The customer proceed to the registers, paid for the merchandise, and then walk toward the front of the store toward a lengthy conveyor belt behind a customer counter. The conveyor belt had large grey bins periodically appearing from the store room. An employee called out a ticket number and the customer received his or her merchandise; a unique shopping experience for its time.

Sharon, seeing an ad in the local paper proclaiming discounts on all jewelry decided they should see what they had to offer. Todd was adamantly against the idea. He still felt that they could possibly afford something bought at a more distinguished establishment. Sitting in the store's parking lot Todd asks, "How would it sound?" "How would what sound?" "How does it sound if someone ask you, 'So where did you get your wedding rings from?' 'Oh we got our weddings rings from Service Merchandise.'" Sharon smiles as the two sit in Todd's orange Mercury Capri, "Todd. I don't care where the rings come from. It's not about the size of the diamond or where we get them from. You know our budget is limited. A ring from here is just fine. The ring is just a symbol of our love which can't be measured in dollars." Todd reluctantly follows Sharon into the store where they are greeted by an employee who asks the couple if they have ever shopped there before. Sharon grasps a clip board and walks over to the jeweler section. Unlike the rest of the store, the jewelry counter was actually manned by an employee.

Sharon and Todd approach the glass cases. An employee asks them, "Is there something I could help you with today?" Sharon replies, "Yes. We're a wedding ring set." The woman behind the counter says, "Oh that's wonderful. Congratulations. Do you know if you would like gold or silver?" Todd looks at Sharon, "Gold?" Sharon replies back to the woman, "Gold would be good." The women walks down the counter a few feet and starts to slide a door open as she pulls out a tray of rings, "Here. I think you might like these." Sharon and Todd walk over to the tray of rings now on top of the glass counter. They peer over the shiny glittering display of rings. The women ask, "Are you looking for a plain band or something with a design? Do you want them matching?" Sharon looks over at Todd as he says, "I'd prefer something plain. What about you?" Sharon looks back at the woman, "I think well go with something plain and something that is a set. We'd like them to match." As Sharon responds back to the women Todd points to a wedding band set, "What about this one? What do you think?" The woman behind the counter pulls out the ring set from the black felt background. Sharon holds the engagement ring in her palm. It was a plain gold band with a single diamond setting. Sharon smiles as she holds the rings in her hand. "I like it. I think they're beautiful." The woman behind the counter replies, "We have lay-away as well." Sharon looks over at the woman, "How much are they?" The woman replies, "We have a sale this week which will make the set very affordable."

Sharon and Todd look at each other for some time as Sharon breaks the silence, "I like them. Let's get these ones." Todd responds, "Are you sure Sharon. Are you sure you want your wedding ring from here?" Sharon responds instantly, "Yes, yes. I'm sure." Todd grimaces knowing he won't win the battle, "OK, but I'm going to get you something bigger and better after we get married, maybe for our tenth anniversary." Sharon smiles back at Todd, "We'll see. We'll just have to see."

It was Christmas Eve, 1985 around 3:00 in the afternoon. Sharon and Todd were sitting on the family room's love seat in Sharon's home. Todd went down onto one knee in front of Sharon, "This is your last chance to say no." Sharon laughed. Todd smiled and said, "Sharon, will be my wife, will you marry me?" Sharon replied, "YES." Todd stands and sits back down next to Sharon as they kiss.

Sharon and Todd's twenty-fifth anniversary was quickly approaching. Just as Todd had done numerous times in the past; at the fifth year, tenth year, fifteenth year, twentieth, and now the twenty-fifth he ask Sharon the same question, "How about we go out and buy you a bigger diamond ring. How about we trade up that Service Merchandise ring with something a bit more upscale?" Just as she had done all those times before, Sharon smiled, grasp his hand in hers, and looked him in the eye saying, "I don't want another ring. This one. This ring is all that I need. It means more to me than any size diamond. It reminds me of us and who we are and how far we have come together." I suspect I will hear those same words from Todd at our thirtieth, thirty-fifth, and so on. I'm sure Todd will not be surprised by my response, the ring remains a symbol of our love, a value that is unquantifiable.

Section Three
Married to the Navy

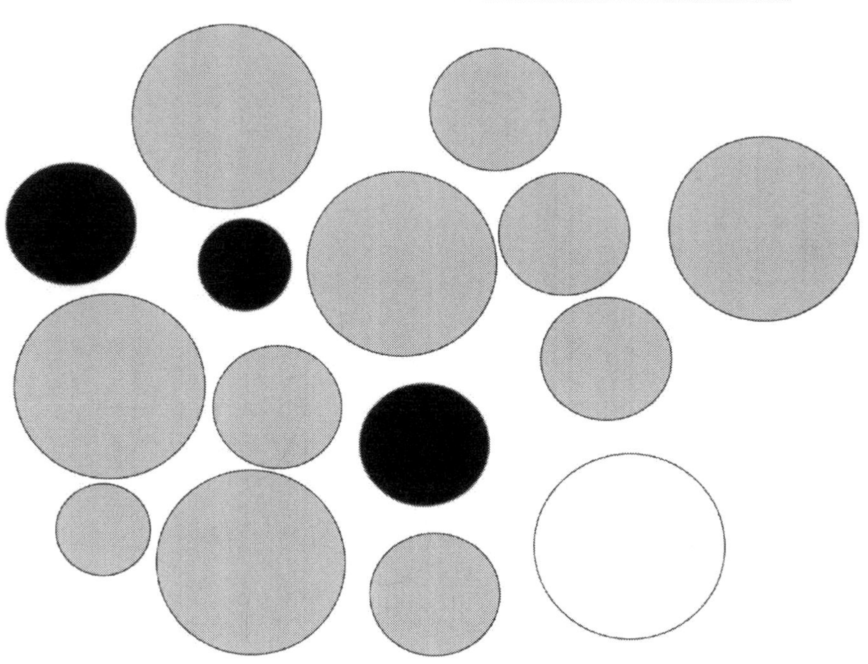

Seurat Dot Eight
A Wedding and a Honeymoon; The Navy Way

It was the middle of December 1987 when Sharon and Todd were married. Sharon was a senior in college and would graduate in May of 1988. Todd was a college senior and a midshipman. As a midshipman, he needed to complete a cruise before he could be commissioned in the Navy. The cruise was scheduled for June of 1988. Knowing this, Sharon and Todd planned for a December wedding. The timing was such that it would be between semesters and would afford them time for a honeymoon.

It wasn't long before their plans for a December wedding would be affected. Todd returned from a meeting with his midshipman advisor, "The Lieutenant told me he had a good deal for me." "What do you mean?" "Well, you know he had worked it so that I'd be on a supply ship in June." "Right?" "He told me today that a spot opened up on a brand new guided missile cruiser." "So....What does that mean?" "Well, it means it would be a heck of a lot more exciting for one, but it also means I'd now leave in December." "Is that going to affect our wedding date?" "No, not our wedding date.....Just our honeymoon." "Where do you have to go?" Todd hesitates, "Well, that's another thing..... I'll be flying out to Australia. I pick up the ship in Sydney. I'll ride the ship back to Hawaii then fly back home." Sharon sarcastically replied, "I see at least it will be a great honeymoon for you."

This was just another military spouse life lesson for Sharon. The lesson that the military gave orders and she just gave opinions; she couldn't change the military orders. Sharon knew that her opinion also affected Todd. She knew it often put Todd at odds with what would be or could be better for his career. A balance that he would often need to strike.

The wedding was conducted in the typical Catholic tradition and was held at Sharon's childhood church, Saint John Fisher. On the evening of their wedding day the weather was bitter cold, there was a biting wind, and of course a light snow. The church altar was lined with poinsettias of every color and size. The wedding party processed up to the altar and assumed their positions on each side. The wedding song begins to play as Sharon with her father by her side walks down the aisle. Sharon couldn't believe the sight that was in front of her; the bridesmaids on one side the groomsmen on the other and of course Todd standing off to the side in his midshipman uniform. Sharon says to herself, "I can't believe the day is finally here."

The service at the Church ended. Todd and Sharon kissed for the first time as husband and wife. Several of Todd's fellow Midshipmen from his unit had gotten together and formed a traditional "sword arch" down the last portion of the churches main aisle. As the couple approached, the Midshipmen drew their swords and placed them in the air to form an arch. Todd and Sharon processed down the archway. As Sharon walked past the last Midshipmen she was given the inaugural sword spank followed by the utterance of the words, "Welcome to the Navy!"

At the reception hall the traditional toast were given, speeches made, the first dance was done, and the last slice of Baked Alaska cake was served. With the music still playing loudly and friends and family dancing, Todd and Sharon slipped out the back of the reception hall driving the orange Mercury Capri back to Sharon's house.

Sharon packed away her wedding gown and changed into more comfortable clothes. She picked up her overnight bag as Todd flung his green sea bag over his shoulder and headed back out to the car. Seeing the sea bag was a reminder to Sharon of just how short their honeymoon together would be.

"Our marriage was tested from the very beginning. Todd had orders to depart just two days after our wedding. We were married on a Saturday and he left in the early morning hours on Monday." Todd's orders called for him to depart from O'Hare airport. They decided it was best to stay up at the O'Hare Marriott, minutes from the airport.

Sharon and Todd arrived at the hotel, checked into their single room, placed their luggage on the dresser and embraced. "The day was a blur. It just flew by" Sharon couldn't believe how exhausted she was.

For Sharon, Sunday brought what would be a new reality to her life. No longer was it just talk. No longer was it something off in the future. It was happening to her here and now. Sharon often refers to it as, "impending departure depression". The experience of knowing your spouse will be leaving, wanting to spend every moment together, but knowing your separation is inevitable, there's nothing you can do to stop it.

For a couple who were known for their maturity and detailed planning, Sharon and Todd found themselves at a loss, unsure of how to spend their first day together as husband and wife. They resorted to what they knew best. They fell back on what any good Chicago couple would do on a wintery Sunday. They went to a small convenience store, purchased a bag of tortilla chips, a can of cheese dip, headed back to the room, and watched the Bears game on television while sharing a bowel of nachos.

Sunday evening was a splurge. Sharon was familiar with the hotel and knew there was an upscale restaurant on the first floor called "The Konaki." The realization that Todd would be heading out in less than twelve hours was beginning to become a reality.

The next morning they packed up their things, headed down to the lobby, paid their bill, and walked into the bitter cold dark of the early morning hour. They approached the airport terminals and headed toward the short term parking garage.

They held hands the entire way into the airport terminal, the duffle bag flung over Todd's shoulder. Todd checked the duffle bag at the counter and they headed toward security as Sharon accompanied Todd all the way to the gate.

They sat in the terminal, made some small talk, all the while working to keep back their true emotions. Sharon held back her tears, knowing if she broke down in front of Todd it would make it even harder for him to leave.

The final boarding call was announced across the gates intercom. They stood up, both trying to capture the last few moments together. They kissed, hugged, and said their goodbyes. Todd walked into the gateway, turned, looked over his shoulder, and waved back toward Sharon one last time. Sharon turned to head back to the parking garage, tears beginning to give way to her previously stoic appearance, "I can remember walking through the terminal as fast as I could, tears rolling down my face. I just wanted to get to the car so that I could cry alone, without anyone else around to see me."

Sharon started the car in the airport garage. She wiped away the tears that still flowed down her cheeks. She knew that she had to pull herself together if she was going to drive the dreaded expressway. Sharon hated the expressway driving, a fact that could be crippling to anyone who lived in or around Chicago. In the day's that led up to Todd's departure, he asked Sharon several times, "Are you sure you'll be ok on the expressway?" Sharon was adamant, she would do it, and she would do it herself.

She followed the signs for the exit out of the airport and onto the toll road. All the while sniffling and wiping the tears from her eyes. "I'm coming home from my honeymoon, a married women, but with no husband nearby. I couldn't get over the fact my life was going to be back to normal (before I was married), I'd work full time, sleep in the same bed alone; it was going to be the longest three weeks in my life."

Sharon made it home without incident. She parked the car in her family's driveway. Her eyes blood shot from the crying. Her mother tried to consul her by placing her arm around Sharon. The embrace wasn't enough. She peeled away her mother's caring hand and headed straight back to her bedroom.

Sharon placed a CD into the player, lies atop her bed, as Ben her dog jumps up onto the bed with her. Ben seemingly knows that Sharon is hurting, that she is upset. Sharon reaches toward Ben, pulls him into her arms, the fur on his ears become wet as Sharon's tears land on the dog's head. She gripped Ben tightly, holding him as she tried to regain control of her emotions.

Sharon relayed the irony of the CD that she was listening to, "I realized afterward the CD was Elton John's *Live in Australia with the Melbourne Symphony Orchestra.*" The CD was released in July of 1987, while the music on the CD was recorded live on 14 December, 1986, nearly one year to the date of their wedding.

Seurat Dot Nine
Our First Christmas

Christmas Day, Sharon was spending her first holiday alone. Well, technically not alone, Sharon was with her family but her husband was in Australia.

Sharon tried to enjoy the holiday as best she could, making small talk with family members, all the while thinking about Todd. Later that afternoon, the phone rings. Sharon believes it's just another person wishing her parents well for the holidays. The phone rings once more when Sharon's mother picks up the receiver from the wall. Her mother hears a voice on the other end saying, "Hello?" Todd starts to talk loudly through the receiver thinking that if he did he could be heard more clearly on the other end. "This is Todd." "Oh Todd! Hold on! Hold On! Sharon will be so glad to talk with you!" Sharon's mom calls out to Sharon in the front living room, "Sharon. You need to come to the phone. It's Todd." Sharon races toward the phone in the kitchen and grasp the phone from her mother's hands.

"Todd! Is it you!" "Sharon! Sharon it's me. I'm in Sydney, Merry Christmas!" "Merry Christmas to you." I miss you so much." "I miss you too." The clicking continued and the stack of coins began to dwindle. "I can't talk long. I'm standing here having to throw coins into this phone in order to keep talking with you. I'm almost out of money. Are you doing ok?" Sharon replies, "Yea. I'm fine. I'm doing fine. How are you?" "I'm fine. An Australian couple who were taking a tour of the ship asked me if I'd like to go to the yacht club with them and watch the start of the race. They call the day after Christmas here Boxing Day. It's a pretty big deal I guess." "That sounds great. I'm glad you have something to do." "I just wanted to call and hear your voice before the ship heads out for Hawaii. Hopefully the rest of the time will go by in a hurry. I'll call you when I get into Hawaii." Todd hears a clicking sound in the line… He assumes the clicking sound is an indication that the coins he inserted into the phone were being used up. Todd reaches down for his last coin as he places it in the phone, "I love you Sharon. I miss you." "I love you too……" The phone call abruptly ends.

Sharon places the receiver back on the kitchen wall, abruptly turns, and heads back into her room with tears streaming down her face. She called for Ben and closed the door behind her. She needed Ben, "That dog was the biggest attachment I had to Todd." No one in Sharon's family had ever spent Christmas without their spouse, "It just wasn't something our family was familiar with." Sharon wondered, "Would it get any easier spending time apart?"

One by one Sharon's sisters and her mother periodically came into her bedroom to check on her. Sharon was propped up on the bed, clutching Ben in her arms, tears flowing down her face, and a box of tissues nearby. Sharon's family asked, "Is there anything we can do?" Sharon replied to each in kind, "I just want to be alone." No one knew what to do. No one had experienced this before. All they could do at the time was respect Sharon's desire for privacy and to let her know they were there if she needed them.

Sharon began to fight the feeling of not wanting to be a "downer" on everyone's holiday. She knew she had to pull herself together and put things in perspective. Sharon reached for some tissues, wiped away the tears, sniffled a few times, and petted Ben one last time before she stood up from her bed and made her way back to the kitchen to join the rest of the family.

The weeks dragged by, Sharon did her best at trying to stay busy, "I tried to absorb myself in routine. My socializing was limited to just a few times when I would go out with my family or friends." No one knew what to say, "The country was not at war. The military life style was foreign where I grew up. I felt like I was on an island some times. I had no way of getting a hold of Todd. There was no phone line to the ship, no internet, and email. Just time and distance between the two of us."

The depression and anxiety of Todd's departure soon transformed itself into excitement and anticipation, knowing Todd's return was just days away. "I was so excited the night before his arrival that my mother said to me, 'Sharon, you need to get some rest. You have to be up by 4:00 in the morning.' I know mom. I can't fall asleep. The excitement is just eating me up inside. I'm just too wired to sleep."

Sharon drove the expressways back to the Airport. Smiling and excited to see Todd once again. Sharon drove into the airports parking garage and headed toward the gate to meet the airplane. Sharon hears the gate agent announce the arrival of Todd's plane. Moments pass when suddenly the doors to the gate are opened by an agent. One by one passengers begin to flow through the doorway. Sharon looks on intently, trying to catch a glimpse of Todd's face.

A log jam of passengers began to form at the gate, then, amongst all the faces she sees Todd's. Even though she could see him she wasn't able to make her way through the bodies of people still trying to leave the gate, "I just wanted to push my way through to get to him. I knew that wasn't appropriate, so I waited."

Todd saw Sharon and from that moment on they never took their eyes off one another. Todd weaved himself through the bodies of passenger's intent on making his way to Sharon as quickly as he could.

Finally, after nearly four weeks apart, Todd and Sharon are able to embrace each other once again. It was nearly four weeks since the wedding, nearly four weeks since they last were able to hold each other in their arms, "It was so amazing to feel Todd's arms around me once again. To feel him close to me. Words can't describe how good it felt to have him back."

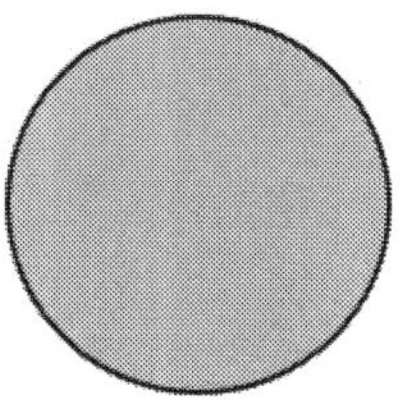

Seurat Dot Ten
First Set of Orders

Sharon and Todd were the last sibling in a family of five. They wanted a larger sized family and knew that waiting wouldn't help matters especially when Todd knew his first couple of years as a student Naval Flight Officer would be dedicated to training and not deployments. Sharon and Todd both graduated in 1988. Sharon was happy that she had gotten her degree but also knew she would have little use for it as a new military spouse and an expectant mother.

With orders now in hand to report to Naval Air Station Pensacola Florida for flight school Sharon and Todd packed up both cars, and headed south early one fall morning. This was the first time that Sharon would ever leave her childhood home not knowing when she would return, or when she would see her parents next.

They arrived in Pensacola in the fall of 1988, driving two cars from Chicago over two days. Sharon always remembered what it felt like on the second day of the drive as they approached the Florida Pan Handle. The temperature steadily increasing with each passing mile. As the temperature climbed Sharon realized that her Chicago fall attire was not going to cut it in the south. She wrestled to remove her jacket and sweater as drove along the highway, peeling off layer after layer, tossing the garments in the back of the car.

The first order of business was to find a place to live. The second, was to find Sharon an OB/GYN. They moved what little they had into a small two bedroom town house about thirty-five minutes from the base where Todd would be stationed. The townhouse was about a fifteen minute walk to the white sandy beaches of Pensacola. After checking in with the base hospital Sharon was given a "non-availability" statement which basically meant she would be allowed to see a doctor "out in town".

Sharon quickly experienced what it was like to belong to this new family, "the Navy family." Sharon was walking the dog outside the townhouse when a women from across the street, living in another unit approaches. The woman introduces herself, "Hello. I noticed you have blue stickers on your car. Are you military?" Sharon replied, "Oh yes." The women asks, "Pilot or NFO?" Sharon immediately replies, "NFO." "Where did you PCS from?" "We were in Chicago. This is our first duty station." "I see you're pregnant. How far along are you?" "I'm due in January." "That's wonderful. I just had our first about six weeks ago. Have you found a doctor?" "Funny you should ask, I'm looking for a doctor now." "Oh are you. Let me tell you my OB was fantastic. He works out of the Pensacola Children's Hospital as well. I really recommend him if you haven't found anyone. You'll be very impressed with the hospital as well." "Thanks so much." Sharon takes the woman's suggestion and sets up her first appointment.

Todd checked into the Training Command and learned that he would be "stashed" for a couple of months, waiting for a class to open up. The days that followed were mostly spent watching Sharon's pregnant belly get larger, and larger.

The first of the New Year arrived, Sharon and Todd had spent their first Christmas together although this time away from family. A few days into the New Year Todd finds out that he'll be starting his Aviation Indoctrination class at the end of the month. Todd hoped that Sharon would deliver before then so that he could be there for her at the house, at least for a while.

It was now early January when Sharon began to experience some "pains". The pains grew closer and closer together, "Todd, I think we should go to the hospital now." Todd grabbed Sharon's bag and they headed off to the hospital where they checked into a birthing room. The OB came into the room and checked on Sharon. "You're defiantly in labor. Let's give it a bit more time though. I think it's best if you go back home for now. Maybe take a walk or do some jumping jacks." The doctor smiles at Sharon. Sharon's face grimaces at the thought she'd have to go home, that it wasn't time yet. The pains she was feeling were intense. Sharon wondered how long it would take. How long the pains would go on for.

After a sleepless and restless night the contractions continued well into the afternoon when Sharon decided it was time to go back to the hospital. Once again, the nurses checked Sharon in and got her settled into a birthing room. The doctor arrived in the room and began to asses Sharon's progress. "Good news. You're going to have that baby today. You're not going back home. You still have a ways to go through but I'll check in on you in a bit." Sharon smiled at the news that she would be giving birth soon as more contractions began to set in. The nurses hook up a monitor to her belly which provided some indication as to the duration of the contractions. The contractions came closer and closer together.

Later that evening, different doctor entered the room. She identified himself as being part of the OB/GYN group and the weekend duty. She made a point at telling Sharon and Todd she specialized in complex births. Sharon was reassured by this fact but hoped she wouldn't be in need of her extra skills. After checking Sharon's progress the doctor says, "Ok. It's not going to be long now. How about we get Dad in a set of scrubs and we'll get you into the operating room." Todd's face appears concerned, "Operating room?" The doctor replies, "Oh yes. Since this is your first we prefer to deliver in the OR just in case. Don't worry. Everything is fine. I don't expect any problems."

Sharon is rolled out of the room headed towards the OR. Todd takes up his position by Sharon's face dressed in green colored scrubs. Todd reassures her that everything is fine and that she's doing a great job.

A soft cry of a new born baby fills the room as the doctor says, "Congratulations, it's a Boy!"

Sharon spent two days in the hospital before being able to bring home their first born. They named their first born Joshua Todd after deciding to use a combination of biblical names and family first names.

As new parents, Sharon and Todd were amazed how much energy could be found in such a cute little baby boy. Todd referred to baby Joshua as the "energizer bunny".

Endless crying and fussing quickly contributed to Sharon's feeling of inadequacy as a mother; nothing seemed to pacify little Joshua. They resorted to various pacifying methods such as; taking long car trips, placing the infant carrier on top the running dryer, and white noise. With nothing seemingly working, their parenting skills in question, they broke out the wind up baby swing. Still officially too young for the contraption but nowhere else to turn and no further tricks up their sleeves, they placed a rolled up bath towel around Joshua's little head to prop him up; Joshua was able to enjoy the swaying back and forth while Todd and Sharon both enjoyed a few minutes of peace.

Regrettably, the success of the swing quickly faded and Sharon had only one more option; to face the pediatrician and fess up to her seeming motherly faults. Sharon brought Joshua into the clinic where she was introduced to her first pediatric medical term; Colic. In none medical terms it means; a baby who never sleeps and instead fills that time with crying. The doctor assured Sharon that she had done everything right and suggested on more possible course of action; changing the formula to a soy based type.

Sharon left the clinic more confident in her motherly abilities and headed directly to the base commissary to pick up a soy formula.

To make matters even more interesting for Sharon, Todd arrived home with news that he was finally assigned a start date for aviation indoctrination training or AI. AI was a six week period where the students endured, numerous written exams, obstacle courses, running, dunking machines, treading water, a one mile swim, and ....

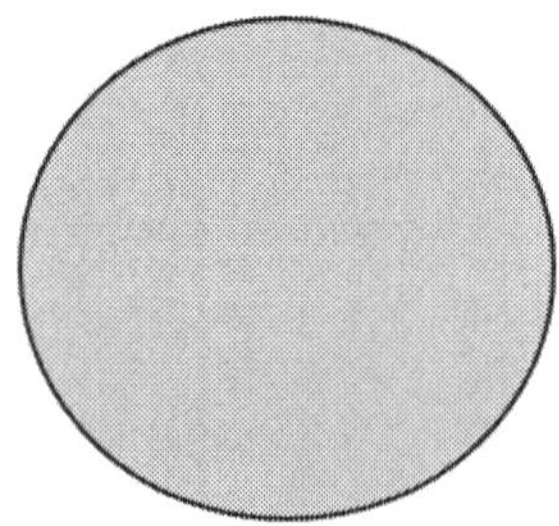

Seurat Dot Eleven
Three Days

One evening towards the end of Todd's training he informs Sharon he needs to attend a three day survival training event. "Sharon, they tell us we'll be heading out for a few days as they teach us some basic survival skills."

"Are you coming back each day?"

"No. They bus us to a location. It will be for three days. Are you going to be OK?"

"Well I don't have a choice, but we'll be fine."

Such was Sharon's way. She quickly compartmentalized her own emotions and provided the appearance of confidence while reassuring Todd at the same time all will be handled on the home front.

Sharon awoke early in the morning, bundled Josh up in his car seat and drove Todd to the base gym where he would meet up with the rest of his class. Sharon kissed Todd and waved goodbye as she began to wonder to herself, "How will I manage. I've only been here for a few months. I hardly know anyone here. I don't have any family nearby. What am I going to do? How will I fill the time?"

"Those three days dragged. I'll be honest, I just wanted to get through them as fast as I could. I took walks with Josh and we even went down to the beach a couple of times. Three days alone felt like it was going to be an eternity."

On the last day of Todd's survival training Sharon pulls together the ingredients for a coffee cake. Sharon realizes, "He's got to be starving after three days in the wilderness and no food to eat."

Sharon places Joshua in his car seat as she sits the newly baked coffee cake on the passenger seat, a fork sitting nearby, and heads back to the base to pick Todd up from his training.

Sharon parks the car and waits anxiously for the buses to arrive. The busses pull up and come to a stop as Sharon steps out of the car, stands by the car door, looking for Todd to appear. Todd makes eye contact and rushes toward her, they embrace, and Todd immediately opens the car and pulls Joshua out of his car seat to hold him in his arms.

Todd smiles when he sees the coffee cake and fork sitting in the passenger seat, "You shouldn't have done this. You have your hands full. I would have been fine."

"I know. But you have to be hungry."

"I won't lie. I'm hungry and this coffee cake is delicious."

Sharon smiles back at Todd, happy to see him content, and even happier knowing the family was back together again.

Seurat Dot Twelve
Choanal Stenosis

The time was late March 1990, Sharon and Todd were expecting their second child. Sharon was in her last trimester, about the eighth month point, when the small family of three arrived in Jacksonville, Florida. Todd's orders to Jacksonville were a short one. They were to stay in Jacksonville for about eight weeks before heading out once again, this time, back to Pensacola Florida, where their journey all began. If the doctors were right, and nature obliged, their second baby would be born in Jacksonville and in enough time for Sharon to recoup before heading out once again. The risk of delivering en route to Pensacola was a real one and one they just as soon not consider at this point.

There is a quaint saying in the Navy that goes, "If the Navy wanted you to have a wife and kids they would have issued them to you in your sea bag." Sharon and Todd had orders, like it or not. Sharon knew she had an option, to stay with her parents until the baby was born while Todd goes it alone. Sharon knew staying with her parents would be easier on Josh and herself. It would have certainly reduced the number of obstetricians she'd have to see. But Sharon chose to stay with Todd throughout the series of short temporary duty assignments.

In the early morning hours on 5 May, 1990, Todd drove Sharon to the local hospital. The sun was now beginning to show itself as they walked into the emergency room. Todd went off to fill out some paperwork while a nurse took Sharon to the delivery floor.

Now, about 0800 in the morning with Todd by her side in the birthing room, he held Sharon's hand as the fetal monitor indicated the onset of yet another contraction. Todd looked at Sharon in an attempt at diverting her attention from the pain and to ensure she would breathe through the duration of the contraction. Sharon squeezed Todd's hand tightly, so tight, that his fingers would nearly turn blue. Todd didn't care how tight she squeezed or what color his fingers turned, he just knew allowing Sharon to do so was in some small way a means of transference of her pain.

About an hour had passed when the doctor once again examined Sharon. This time, the doctor told Sharon it was "time to push." Those three words were music to her ears. Hearing them, Sharon knew the end of labor was in sight. She also knew she could let her body do what it had wanted to do all morning. Instead of breathing through the contractions she could now push through them. From this point on, the doctor orchestrated the remainder of the delivery, telling Sharon when to push and when not to. After several minutes had gone by a soft cry is heard coming from the end of the bed. The doctor clips the umbilical cord, hands the new born over to the nurse who promptly wipes the baby down. The nurse hands the new born over to Sharon, placing the baby briefly on her chest so she could welcome the baby to this world. It was another boy.

After a couple of days recouping from the delivery, it's time to take Sharon home with Josh's new baby brother, Zachariah. Just ten days after Sharon had given birth the family of now four set out once again. They packed up a small U-Haul trailer and began their trek across the Pan Handle to Pensacola.

After a full day of driving, they arrived in Pensacola and checked into the Navy Lodge. The family was assigned one of the older bases houses, now converted into Navy lodging.

Todd's assignment in Pensacola this time, was to "Corry Station", a small adjunct to the main base where he conducted his initial flight training. Sharon and Todd's primary objective after checking into the command was to find housing. Within a day or two, they found an unfurnished apartment just outside the gate of Corry Station. The location was perfect, Todd could ride his bike into work while leaving Sharon full access to the car.

The days that followed were hectic as Sharon and Todd made the rounds with various offices to rapidly set up their temporary home. Sharon and Todd moved the family into the first floor apartment after heading to the local Rent-A-Center. They outfitted the apartment with only the basics. Todd commented, "Sharon was a wiz at starting up electric, cable, and phone services. She could have the family up and running in the matter of hours."

Without the luxury of a full sized crib, Sharon and Todd purchased a three-in-one travel crib. In the simple two bedroom apartment the travel crib worked perfectly. Sharon setup the crib in their bedroom. This way she could feed Zach during the night and not disturb Josh's sleep.

Zach was now about a month old and began to show signs of having his first cold. Because he was so young, Sharon took him into the pediatrician to be seen. The doctor recommended Tylenol to control the low grade fever he was experiencing.

Two days passed, Zach's fever began to get worse and he began to sound congested. Concerned, Sharon immediately brought him back to the doctor.

This time the doctor ordered a chest X-Ray. The X-Ray results were good, his chest was clear. The doctor recommended a cool bath for his fever, continued use of the Tylenol to control the fever, and to bring him back if the fever doesn't break.

Sharon placed Josh in his bed for the night as she returned to the bassinet to give Zach his evening feeding. Sharon was sitting up in the bed holding Zach in her arms as she tried to feed Zach. Something wasn't right; Sharon knew it and Todd knew it. Zach couldn't seem to take the bottle. He'd spit out the formula from his mouth; it would just run down the sides of his cheeks. Sharon tells Todd, "I'm taking him back to the doctor in the morning. He's not right." Todd looks back at Sharon, "Yeah, I definitely agree with you. Something is not right with him."

Sharon starts to shake Todd awake saying, "He's not breathing right. I think he has stopped breathing." Todd replies, "He stopped breathing? What?" Sharon immediately put on a pair of jeans, placed Zach in his car carrier, and headed out the door saying, "He's not breathing right. I'm taking him to the ER now." Todd now more coherent, "Yes. Yes. Go…. Call me when you can. I'll take care of Josh." The base hospital emergency room was just minutes from the apartment.

Sharon rushes into the ER and up to the nurse's station saying, "My baby is not breathing right." Immediately, a nurse standing nearby takes Zach back to the triage area while Sharon provided the intake staff with some basic information. Soon after, Sharon is lead back to the triage room where Zach was lying in the middle of a large adult sized gurney with a pulse/oxygen monitor clipped to his big toe. Sharon quickly realizes that she has the attention of the entire ER staff. The doctor in charge orders an Arterial Blood Gas (ABG) gas lab. The ABG is a measure of how well your lungs are able to move oxygen into your blood.

Sharon comments to the staff, "He's looking a little blue." The staff busily began to run test in an attempt to understand why the oxygen they had running through his nose wasn't doing enough for him. Seconds later, a nurse asks Sharon to leave and have a seat in the waiting room. The nurse asks Sharon as she walks her to the waiting area, "Do you have anyone here with you?" Sharon replies, "No. It's just me. My husband is home with my other son."

Hearing this fact the nurse replies in an insistent tone, "I'll have another nurse come out and sit with you."

The hospital was quiet, there were few people in the ER at the time with the exception of those attending to Zach. Sharon hears Zach crying from behind the double doors leading to the triage area where she had just been moments earlier. The nurse sitting next to Sharon attempts to comfort her by saying, "It's ok that he is crying." Sharon replies in a tearful manner, "At least I know he is alive."

Nearly twenty minutes later Sharon is allowed to see Zach once again. Sharon see's Zach and the ER doctor and in an emotional voice asks, "What's wrong him? What's wrong with my baby?" The ER doctor responds, "We're not exactly sure. We need to send him to Sacred Heart Children's Hospital." Sharon begins to contemplate the fact that she will be taking Zach to yet another hospital when the doctor adds, "We've called for a life flight helicopter. It will be here soon. He NEEDS to be at Sacred Heart, not here." Sharon appears stunned at what the doctor was saying, "What? Life Flight? Why does he need to be life flighted? Why can't he just be taken in an ambulance?" Sharon associates the life flight helicopter with the thought of imminent death. The doctor explains, "He's not stable enough to handle the drive." Sharon responds forcefully, "I'm coming with then." The doctor responds, "I'm sorry Mrs. Kruder but you can't, there isn't room. Are you able to drive?" Sharon answers nervously, "Yes. Yes I can drive." The doctor looks at Sharon and says, "That's best and Mrs. Kruder...... Don't try and beat the helicopter. There's no way you can. Just drive carefully."

The phone on the wall in the apartment rings as the sound of a helicopter can be heard making an approach over the base. Up to this point Sharon was battling her inner emotions. She didn't want to be kicked out of the room yet again. Now, with the nurses and doctors preparing Zach for the flight to Children hospital she says to Todd in an emotionally distraught manner, "Todd, it's me. They are taking my baby. They are taking him on a life flight to Sacred Heart now." Todd can't believe what Sharon is telling him, "They are what? Flying him? How is he?" Sharon replied, "The doctors aren't sure what is wrong with him. He's not stable enough to make the trip in an ambulance. This is the fastest way." Sharon wanted to get back to Zach and not be on the phone any longer than she had to be saying to Todd, "I need to go now. Call Tammie (a close friend) and see if she can take Josh. I will pick you up and we can drive to the hospital together." "Ok. I love you. Hang in there Sharon; I'm sure he'll be fine." Todd knew that these words were simply spoken to keep Sharon's spirits up.

Sharon and Todd arrived at the hospital and made their way to the pediatric intensive care unit. As the couple navigate the many hallways and corridors they find some of the sights familiar as this was the same hospital Sharon gave birth to Joshua just over a year and a half ago.

Once they arrived at the unit a nurse greeted the both of them. Sharon instantly request, "How's my baby? Can I see him?" The nurse politely replies, "Not at the moment. We're in the process of evaluating your son now. It should only be a few more minutes before the doctor can meet with you. Why don't you have a seat in the waiting area? The doctor will be out shortly."

Several minutes pass before a doctor appears in the waiting area, "Mr. and Mrs. Kruder?" Sharon and Todd stand and walk towards the doctor, "Yes." "I'm the doctor that will be taking care of your son. I've evaluated his condition and believe he has what is called Coanal Stenosis." Sharon and Todd appear puzzled by the medical jargon. The doctor continues, "For about the first three months of an infant's life, they are considered to be an obligate nose breather. This means their brains have not yet matured enough to know to use their mouths for breathing, as well as their nose. When Zachary got a cold it swelled the inner membranes of his nose. In essence it was suffocating him, depriving him of oxygen. So you can see how the results can be tragic and can be a contributing factor in Sudden Infant Death Syndrome (SIDS)" Sharon asks, "So what do you do about it?" The doctor replies, "Well, in this case I recommend we insert tubes into his nasal cavity. The tubes will keep the passageway open. This should help him breathe and get his oxygen levels back up to where they should be." "We'll need to have you both fill out some forms and we get Zachery scheduled for the procedure."

Still wearing his scrubs and cap he approached grinning, "Mr. and Mrs. Kruder. The surgery went great. Zachary did wonderfully. I was able to insert the tubes just like we discussed." Sharon jumps to her feet, "When can I see him?" "He's being brought into ICU right now. Once they have him stable I'm sure you two can see him."

Sharon will never forget what her baby looked like lying on a small bed. One toe was covered by a shiny orange light, his arms taped to foam covered boards, oxygen running into his nose, and wires attached to his tiny chest. He just lied there as the beeping from the monitors filled the room. Sharon gently ran the back of her hand across his tiny cheeks, hands, and feet. She would have given anything just to hold her baby once again.

Todd and Sharon cycled back and forth to the hospital. They still had Josh to worry about and Todd had his classwork to manage. On a typical day Sharon would drop Josh off at the day care center first thing in the morning and then head into the hospital to be with Zach. Todd rode his bike onto the base and when the day was done he would ride the bike over to the day care center and pick up Josh. The day care providers always smiled when they would pull his things from the cubby. Typically there would be a jacket, change of clothes and of course, a matching bike helmet. Todd strapped josh into the bike seat and they headed off back to the apartment.

Sharon returned to the apartment around 6:00 in the evening and Todd would drive back to the hospital where he would spend much of the evening. They would do this shuffling again and again for about a week.

During this time Todd became worried that he wasn't going to be able and keep up with the class so he asked to see the Class Instructor, a Navy Lieutenant. He sat in an office chair across from the Lieutenant and explained the situation. Todd told him all about Zach's condition, "I'm concerned I won't be able to keep up with the class. I think I need to roll back a class." The Lieutenant looks at Todd after scanning a grade report sheet and snaps back the following response, "I don't see why. You haven't failed anything yet." Todd, surprised by the comment replies, "Yes Sir. I understand but I'm concerned I won't be able to keep up." The Lieutenant leans across the desk and looks at Todd, "Let's wait and see. You're doing well right now. If you need to roll back a class we can do that. For now let's just see how it goes." "Ok Sir. Thank you for the time."

Zach was brought back home after spending two weeks at the children's hospital and the having the tubes inserted into his nose. Sharon was taught infant CPR and was trained on how to clean the tubes periodically using a small electric vacuum pump. Sharon passed on this knowledge to Todd and the couple continued their busy lives and raising their two children.

Nearing the end of Todd's training at Corry Station they discovered Zach's condition would change their original itinerary. Zach required one more visit to the ENT in order to be cleared for overseas travel. This resulted in an ORD MOD or orders modification resulting in a one month delay. Happy that Zach was well on his way to a full recovery Sharon and Todd began to process through all the requirements needed to head overseas. Unbeknownst to the couple, the change in plans meant their dog, Ben, could no longer be sent overseas with them.

With Todd's class complete and a couple of weeks before Zach's next ENT appointment they drove back to Chicago. While in Chicago visiting family, Sharon's sister, graciously volunteered to watch Ben. Sharon's sister had small children herself and Ben was all about small children. It was a very amenable relationship.

Regrettably, Ben, the dog Sharon used as a Kleenex when Todd made his first departure right after they married, the dog who sat with Sharon during baby feeding times, and the dog who could make Josh and Zach laugh like their little bellies were going to bust ate several ears of corn from the trash and was euthanized.

Seurat Dot Thirteen

¡Bienvenido!

The day for Sharon, Todd, Joshua, and Zachariah began early in Philadelphia. The family checked out of the hotel and took a shuttle to the airport. Once at the airport, they proceeded to the Military Airlift Command (MAC) check-in counter. Their bags, which contained everything they had lived with for the past six months, were checked and disappeared from sight. The family of four were confirmed on the "rotator", a wide bodied jet leased by the defense department for the sole purpose of moving personnel assigned overseas. Todd had received his first set of orders as a Naval Flight officer to Rota Spain and a squadron called VQ-2 or Fleet Air Reconnaissance Squadron Two.

The family headed to the airports United Services Organization (USO) to wait out the nearly six hours before the scheduled departure. After multiple diaper changes, bottle feedings, peek-a-boo games, and strolls through the airport; the time had come for the family to board the aircraft.

Their almost twelve hour journey was now coming to an end as the shades on the windows were raised and the flight crew made their final preparations for landing. Sharon looked out through the plane's window as the plane descended. Sharon turned toward Todd saying, "Is this it? Is this Rota?" Sharon was watching farm land and small homes pass by under the aircraft.

Todd peers out the window to have a look for himself, "I guess so. Why?" Sharon replies, "Where are the buildings? Where's the city at?"

Given Sharon's background she was caught off guard by the lack of city buildings and infrastructure. Simply by coincidence, Sharon had taken four years of High School Spanish and had seen numerous photos of Madrid and Seville; although not many of the southern portion of the country. Rota, a small coastal town in the Province of Cádiz was located near the larger city of Jerez de la Frontera in the south of Spain.

The plane settled in over the runway as the plane touched down on Spanish soil. Sharon was now nearly 4000 miles away from her family in Chicago. The plane taxi's toward a white two story building with an outstretched blue awning. On the ground was a painted sign which read, "Welcome to NAS Rota, Spain."

Sharon and the family followed the rest of the passengers into the terminal building where new arrivals were greeted by their command sponsors. Several minutes pass by when a Lieutenant introduces himself to Todd as his "fill-in" sponsor. The actual sponsor was a female Lieutenant who was called out on a deployment at the last minute.

The sponsor helped Todd with their bags and graciously offered to take them to his house on base for lunch. Tired from the long journey, Todd's reply was nearly automatic, "Oh, that would be great. Thank you." After driving on base for several minutes they begin to approach the base housing. Sharon unexpectedly retorts, "This looks like the slums of Chicago. Look at that place over there with all the garbage sitting outside." The sponsor looked back over his shoulder at Sharon saying, "Oh that over there. That's my house, welcome to USA Housing." Todd instantly cringed at the impression Sharon just made, realizing for the next three years, the squadron was their new extended family.

Seurat Dot Fourteen Deployment

The Kruder family eventually settled in housing located just outside the Fuentebravia base gate. They rented a newly constructed townhouse owned by a Spanish Navy Officer. The experience of living in this European style home was eye opening, it would take some time to adjust to the culture.

Todd settled into his squadron and began the rigorous training track to become a qualified navigator. Todd recalls an Intel Officer at the squadron telling him in a sarcastic tone, "If your spouse ask you where you are going tell them you are going to the Quick Mart." Todd couldn't believe it. He had a hard time thinking Sharon would ever believe him. Besides, Sharon would probably think something was wrong when Todd didn't return for weeks on end. Sharon would have to tolerate numerous deployments, many at the last minute. Sharon lived with the fact of not knowing where Todd was going or what he would be doing.

About two months had now gone by when Todd received word from the Squadron Operations department he would be going on his first deployment; during which he would be expected to fully qualify as a Navigator. Sharon insisted on being at the departure. Todd drove the car to the terminal. The couple unstrapped Josh and Zach from their car seats and headed into the terminal. Several of the crew had already arrived including the "fill-in" sponsor and his wife. The call went out through the terminal to board the airplane. Family members began to hug and kiss each other goodbye. Sharon wraps her arms around Todd, they kiss, and say their goodbyes. Todd kneels down in front of Josh to say goodbye, "Dad will be back soon. Take care of your Mom for me." Todd kiss Zach and Josh goodbye, stands, and grips his green helmet bag. Sharon notices a couple standing off to the side and the wife in tears. There Sharon stood, Josh by her side, Zach in her arms, being left in a foreign country for some unknown amount of time, and not a tear flowing. You can imagine her surprise to see a "seasoned" couple who had likely less than six months left on their orders crying in her husband's arms. Sharon commented, "It's true, the deployments never get easier. The goodbyes are still painful. You just suck it up and deal with it. I wasn't going to break down in front of my kids. They needed to know when dad leaves, mom can handle things. They need to have some sense of parental stability; both emotional, and physical. That's what I tried to provide."

There would many, many more goodbyes, more last minute departures. Sharon, now pregnant with their third child, recalls another time. This time the family was now in the "old base housing", the family just settled down at the dinner table to eat when suddenly the phone on the wall rings. Todd picks up the phone as a voice on the other end says, "Lieutenant Kruder?" "Yes." "This is the Squadron Duty Officer. I've been directed to call you. You'll be leaving tonight." Todd hesitates responding as he runs the thought through his mind and all that comes with it. He replies, "Ok. Can you tell me if I need a small bag or a big bag?" The voice on the other end of the phone pauses, "I'd make it a big bag." The difference between the sizes of the bag meant either days deployed or weeks deployed.

Todd sat back down at the dinner table. Sharon knew what the phone call meant, "So, when do you have to leave?" Todd looks at Sharon and the two boys saying, "I got about an hour before I need to go." Sharon replies, "So is it a small bag or a large bag?" Todd smiles back at Sharon as he replies, "The SDO said to plan on a big bag this time." The conversation then turned toward the boys and what antics they were up to as well as what they did during the day. The family continued to eat, cleaned their dishes, and packed Todd's bag. Before leaving he got on the floor with the boys to play with them one more time. He kissed the boys goodbye, stood up and gave Sharon a hug before leaving yet again.

Seurat Dot Fifteen
Leaving My Babies

Sharon and Todd were now midway through their tour in Rota and living on base in the "Old Spanish Housing". No longer did they have to go on base to make a phone call or walk down to the local pay phone. The old base housing came fully equipped with all the modern conveniences, a phone, washing machine, dryer, oil burning furnace, and cork floors. A white picket fence surround the back yard with plenty of room for Josh and Zach to ride their push cars and even enough room for the "little tykes" log cabin. Routine became Sharon's mantra. The children grew to expect there would be; outside playtime, nap time, reading time, and in the evenings, bath and movie time.

Sharon, having been pregnant twice already knew the signs. She scheduled an appointment at the Naval Hospital on base with the OB/GYN department. She went in and confirmed what she had been feeling. She was pregnant once again. Sharon had come home and decided to break the news to Todd over dinner. Todd smiled as Sharon told him the news, "It must be something in the water" as Sharon and Todd laugh.

A couple of more deployments passed by as Sharon's belly grew larger and larger. Sharon was now entering her second trimester of the pregnancy. Todd recently returned from a detachment and was told by the Ops department he was up for a "good deal". "Good deals" normally meant, a trip state side. It was a great opportunity and he jumped at the chance.

Todd left early to start the pre-flight and planning with the pilots. Later that morning Sharon receives a phone call from the OB/GYN doctor. "The results from your Alpha-Fetoprotein (AFP) test came back abnormal. Since this is the second abnormal finding we need to have an amniocentesis performed. Unfortunately, due to the war, the only option we have is to send you state side, to Bethesda. We'll need you to come in and pick up your records. The admin folks here will make all the arrangements for you."

Sharon nervously hangs up the phone with the doctor. Her thoughts turn immediately toward Josh and Zach. Knowing Todd was leaving for the states and would be gone for two weeks, "Who will take care of my babies?" Sharon calls her close friend Tammie and explains what the doctor told her, "What I'm I going to do Tammie? Todd's gone for two weeks." Tammie asks, "Have you called the President of the Spouses club yet to see if she has any ideas?" "No, I don't know who she is." Tammie knew her and in fact the president of the spouse club was a close neighbor, "Let me call her and see what she can do."

Ten minutes later the phone in the house rings and Sharon answers, "Hello?" It was the president of the spouses club. "I want to call the CO's wife and relay what is going on. Are you ok with that?" Within an hour of their discussion Sharon receives phone call from the CO's wife directly, "Todd's been taken off the flight. He'll be on his way back home soon." Sharon hesitates responding as she fears Todd will be upset having missed an opportunity. Sharon responds, "Thank you." "If there is anything else we can do, don't hesitate calling me."

In the meantime, Todd passes by the Assistant Squadron Duty Officer (ASDO), he hears his name being called out, "Lieutenant Kruder, Lieutenant Kruder!" Todd turned back around and headed over to the ASDO, "What's up?" "Sir, the Commanding Officer (CO) needs to see you now." "The CO? What for do you know?" "Sorry Sir, I don't although he said it was urgent."

Todd entered the CO/XO spaces where he was greeted by one of the yeoman. "Lieutenant Kruder. The Skipper would like to see you." "Sure thing." "Wait just a minute Sir." "No problem." The yeoman disappeared into the CO's office and emergent a few seconds later. The Skipper shouts, "Lieutenant Kruder come on in here!" Todd walked up to the desk where the Skipper was sitting behind. "Lieutenant Kruder. I understand Sharon is expecting?" "Yes Sir, that's correct." "Well I just got a call from my wife." "Yes Sir?" "Evidently Sharon needs to be sent back to the states for some testing. You've got two little ones at home as well?" "Yes Sir." "I've already called the Opso. I've taken you off the flight schedule today. You need to take care of your family right now. Go across the hall to Admin and drop a leave chit. Take whatever time you need." "But what about the flight this morning?" "Like I said, I've taken you off the flight schedule. You have more important things to take care of." "Yes Sir, understood Sir."

Todd arrived home seeing Sharon visibly upset. Sharon began to explain what had happened and what the results of the blood work revealed. More importantly, what the results could mean in terms of birth defects. The possibilities ran the gamut. Of course Sharon focused on only the most severe possibilities, "How are we going to take care of a bay like that? We have two small children already? How are they going to be affected? What kind of quality of life will they have?" Todd looks at Sharon, "What are you suggesting? Are you thinking terminating the pregnancy?" Sharon and Todd were both raised in Catholic faith, a faith that staunchly opposed the act of abortion. Todd tries to refocus Sharon's thoughts, "Let's not jump to any conclusion just yet. You said the blood test is not always accurate. Let's wait and see what the doctors at Bethesda say."

Sharon becomes more emotional as she tries to comprehend how the couple will manage the evolution of her going back to the states, "How Josh and Zach be taken care of." Sharon's maternal instincts run deep. She wouldn't let anyone or anything get in between her and her babies. It was nearly unimaginable for Sharon to think she would be apart from them saying to Todd, "You're the one that leaves, not me." Todd replies, "We'll work it out. Trust me. The kids will be just fine with me."

The day of the rotator Todd submitted leave for the next two weeks and drove Sharon to the terminal. The "rotator" passenger airplane was already sitting on the tarmac. Sharon took her paper work up to the counter and checked her bag. Because of her medical status she was guaranteed a seat. Todd knew his leave chit wouldn't afford them any special treatment. He'd be traveling "Space-A". He also knew that the MAC requirement for seats meant he'd need three. He walked over to the counter as Sharon was watching the kids. "Pardon me. Do you have anything leaving for the states in the next couple of days?" The person behind the counter looks over at a schedule, "Sorry Sir. I don't see anything on the schedule. I'd call back though. There are always flights being added. Do you have our number?" "Thanks. Yea I have it." "Be sure to sign up for Space-A. If there is a flight you'd want to be higher up on the list. The sooner you signup the better." "Ok, I'll do that. Thanks." Todd signs himself, Josh, and Zach up for Space-A then heads back toward Sharon. "What were you doing?" "I was just checking to see if they had any flights back to the states." "Well do they?" "No." Sharon's smile turns into a frown. "Don't you worry; the kids and I will be just fine." "I know you will be. I've never left them before; it's very hard for me." The announcement to board comes across the PA system as passengers begin to funnel through the security check point and walk out to the stairs leading up to the awaiting aircraft. Sharon's eyes begin to fill with tears as she hugs Josh and Zach goodbye. "Call us when you get into Philadelphia." "I will." Sharon and Todd hug one last time as Sharon heads out toward the aircraft.

That evening after Todd fixed the children some dinner he reached into his pocket and pulled out the phone number to the MAC terminal. With the children playing in the background he lifts the phone receiver from the wall and dials the number. A women answers. "Yes, this is Lieutenant Kruder. I was in earlier today and signed up for Space-A. Do you have anything heading back to the states by chance?" "No Sir. I'd recommend you call back tomorrow." "Ok. Thanks."

Sharon's family pulled together rallying to her side. Sharon's brother paid for her sister to fly out to Washington D.C. and to meet Sharon's flight. There, in D.C. her sister by her side they paid for a taxi and headed to Bethesda Naval Hospital. Still, holding the small suitcase Sharon packed the day before in Rota, they headed up to the OB/GYN floor of the hospital where she would have the procedure.

After the procedure Sharon approached the person behind the clinics front desk, "Excuse me. Can I borrow your phone to call for a taxi?" The women responds, "Where are you headed?" "Alexandria?" "Oh, that's close by where I live. You don't need to worry yourself about a taxi. I'll take you there myself." Sharon and her sister arrive in Alexandria, staying at Sharon's - sister's -husband's brother's house while she waited to hear back from the hospital.

Sharon recalls the story Todd often tells of his experience:

The next morning after the kids had eaten their breakfast and had already been out to play in the back yard Todd calls the terminal. "Yes, do you have anything added to the flight schedule?" Todd was anticipating a negative reply so he was shocked to hear, "Yes Sir. We have a flight this afternoon. It's going right into Philadelphia." "Philly? Are you sure?" "Yes Sir. It's a rotator for the local Construction Battalion." "That's great news. Do you expect there will be some open seats?" "Yes Sir. There probably will be." "Ok, thank you."

Todd's excitement grew over the possibility of being able to bring Sharon her babies back. Now he had to figure out how to execute the plan. How would he let Sharon know? How would he get to the terminal? How would they get from Philly to Bethesda? What would he need to pack? How many bottles would he need for Zach? How many outfits? Diapers? One thing was for sure he was determined to bring Sharon her babies. He was determined to be there when Sharon needed him.

Todd communicated his plans to his best friend in the squadron. "If Sharon should call let her know I'm on my way to Philly with the kids."

Todd checked in at the counter for Space-A as the terminal building filled with CB's anxious to get back home. They had been deployed to the "med" for nearly six months. Todd thinks to himself, "Great. I can be on an airplane full of rough and tough guys. Here I am holding a baby and a toddler. What an impression."

The plan began to be boarded by the CB's. As the final few exited the terminal the MAC clerk began to call out the Space-A list. There was no guarantee. Todd wasn't even certain where he and the kids were on the list. The names were called as Todd waited patiently, "Kruder, Todd; Kruder, Joshua; Kruder, Zachariah." Todd leaps up from his chair, gathers his things, places them in the diaper bag and heads to the ticket counter, holding Zach and Josh in trail. He receives his boarding passes and anxiously heads out toward the airplane, uncertain of what adventure he is about to undertake.

Todd walks into the cabin of the airplane, the two children in tow. The plane is filled with the loud voices of the men from the battalion. A stewardess greats Todd as he heads down the aisle in search of his seat. The stewardess smiles at the sight of the children, "Here, let me help you get settled." The stewardess helped Todd with the boys and stowed his bag in the overhead bin.

The cabin door closed as the engines began to whirl. Soon they were taxing to the active runway. The whirl of the engines increased in pitch as the airplane began to race down the runway, the landing gear were raised as the pilots climbed to altitude. There was no inflight movie or entertainment. Just dad, a few books, and a few toys to keep the kids occupied. Zach began to fuss about two thirds into the flight. The stewardess approached Todd, "Is there anything I can get you?" Todd recalled Sharon would often give the children apple juice during the day. "An apple juice in the bottle would be great." The stewardess returns moments later with a completely filled bottle of apple juice. It worked, Zach was comforted by the juice and was once again quiet, a welcome reprieve.

Zach finished the bottle and was content for the time being. The pilots announce they are beginning their descent into Philly. The airplane begins to descend; Zach and Josh begin to complain about their ears. The change in cabin pressure causing their inner ears to ache. Todd explains to Josh how to valsalva; an act of pinching the nose between your fingers, leaning your head back, and then blowing through your nose while keeping your mouth closed. This helps to equalize the pressure and often leads to your ears popping. This worked for Josh who was old enough to follow instructions. Zach was another matter. Todd knew that swallowing was also helpful. He could see that Zach was in pain. Todd waves down the stewardess, "Can I help you?" "Yes, can you give me a bit more apple juice please?" "Certainly. Would you like me to fill the bottle again?" "Yes, that would be great." The stewardess returns with another bottle filled to the brim with apple juice. Todd holds Zach in his lap as he begins to suck on the bottle. "It's working." Zach is no longer pulling at his ears.

The aircraft continues on its descent. The landing gear is extended. The plane begins to shack and vibrate as ground effect begins to set in. Zach drops the now empty bottle to the cabin floor. Todd and Josh are strapped in for the landing. Todd begins to bounce Zach on his lap to entertain him in the last few minutes of the flight. Todd can see the city lights through the oval shaped passenger windows. As the whirl of the engines rise and fall with the throttle movement Todd suddenly feels a warm liquid on his pants. Todd looks down at his Khaki uniform pants to see that Zach had given back the bottle of apple juice and then some. The warm apple juice vomited from Zach's mouth immediately absorbed into Todd's trousers and the lower half of his shirt. The plan lands and heads into the awaiting gate. Todd realizes that he must wait for the CB's to disembark before he was willing to try and maneuver the kids and his newly baptized pair of pants. Of course each and every CB that passed the aisle peered down at the family and snickered. The smell of vomit filled the surrounding seats.

As the last of the CB's disembarked a stewardess rushes over to Todd and provides him a towel to try and absorb the liquid that remained. He thanked the stewardess for her help, gathered up the kids, and threw the diaper bag over one shoulder as he carried Zach in his arms.

They passed by the cockpit and the stewardess who simply smiled and waved. Todd walks through the gate exit to find 30 or forty USO volunteers holding "Welcome Home" banners for the CB's. Their faces became shocked by the sight of this Navy Lieutenant, holding baby in one hand, a diaper bag over his shoulder, and the hand of a toddler. They were even more shocked by the sight of this Lieutenant who looks like he had been through his own battle, covered in apple juice vomit. Todd smiled back at the gracious volunteers and headed quickly out the terminal.

He arrived at the baggage claim, paid a dollar for a luggage cart, and piled on their bags as they came off the carousel. Todd placed Zach in the front of the cart while he asked Josh to watch out for him as he grabbed the bags. Todd's plan now was to get to a hotel for the night and regroup in the morning. He also wanted to contact Sharon who should still be at her sister's brother in laws house in Alexandria. Fortunately, he had the number to the house where she was staying. He pushed the luggage cart over to a bank of pay phones, asked Josh to stay close as Zach who was simply siting in between the metal sides of the carts seat.

Todd places some change in the pay phone and dials the number he had for Sharon. An unknown voice on the other end says, "Hello?" Todd replies, "Yes. My name is Todd Kruder. I believe my wife Sharon is staying with you right now?" "Oh yes. Yes. Hold on just a minute and let me get her for you. Just a minute." A few seconds later Todd hears Sharon pick up the phone, "Hello?" "Sharon, it's me. How are you?" "I'm fine. Where are you?" "We're in Philly." "Philly! Are you kidding me. Are the kids with you?" "Of course they are. What? Do you think I'd leave them behind?" "I can't believe it. I can't believe that you flew them all the way out here. How did you get a flight?" "I called the terminal. They just so happen to have a flight taking the CB's back. It was a straight shot to Philly. Pretty good huh?" "I'd say so." Just then a strange man approaches Todd and taps him on the shoulder, "Excuse me Sir?" Todd, surprised by the tap on the shoulder, immediately turns top face the stranger as he sets eyes on Josh still standing nearby. "Yes?" "I just thought you'd like to know your baby is throwing up all over the floor." "What?" Todd looks down at the luggage cart to find Zach bent over form the waist sitting in the carts child seat, vomit streaming down to the floor below. "Sharon. I have to go. Zach just got sick. I'll give you call from the hotel. Ok?" "OK. You go take care of them and I'll talk with you later."

Todd arrives at the hotel, checks in, heads up to the room, and immediately fills the bath tub with water. He undresses Zach and scrubs him from head to toe, then dresses him for bed. Josh followed suit. Once the kids were finally tucked in Todd showered and rinsed out his uniform from the vomit that was now dried into the fabric. He had made it.

Sharon and her sister immediately make plans of their own to meet Todd in Philly. Sharon's sister's brother-in-law took the two to Union Station early the next morning where they boarded a train and headed back to Philly. Sharon was thrilled, she would soon be reunited with her babies.

Sharon and her sister arrive at the hotel, just as Sharon had planned. There was a knock on the hotel room door. Todd opened the door to the room and there was Sharon, smiling ear to ear. Happy to see Todd and to have her babies back. She quickly hugged Todd and then raced over to Josh and Zach. Josh hugged his mom then something unexpected happened, Zach pulled away and headed toward Todd. Sharon visibly upset says, "What? Have you forgotten your mommy already? I can't believe you won't give me a hug?" Todd eases Sharon's emotions, "I'm sure he's just a bit confused by all the traveling. Besides, I think he has a small fever. I gave Zach some children's Tylenol this morning. He's probably a bit under the weather is all. They know who their mommy is, don't think that they don't."

The family now united once again make plans for the days ahead as they await the test results. They rent a minivan at the airport and drive back to Alexandria where they would stay at a local hotel. Sharon's sister returned back to her own family. In another sign of family support, Sharon's mother and father drove from Chicago to Washington D.C. to be with her.

The waiting seemed to be endless. Time was taken up by visiting a children's museum in D.C., walking through a local Toys-R-Us, or simply walking a local mall.

From the hotel room, Sharon called the hospital multiple times a day asking if they had the results back from the procedure. Sharon was met with the same response, "No Ma'am. Nothing has come back from the lab."

It was later in the afternoon when Sharon once again made her phone call only this time she wasn't greeted with the usual response. This time she was told to stay on the line for the doctor. Sharon's nerves ratcheted up as she waited for the results. Sharon thought to herself, "This can't be good news. Something was wrong. Something is wrong with her baby." Then a male voice on the other end of the phone says, "Mrs. Kruder?" Sharon's nerves become twisted as she waits for the news. Todd, standing by her side quickly shuffles the children into the outer room to watch TV. Todd places his hand on Sharon's shoulder in support for whatever news she may hear. "Mrs.

Kruder, I've got the results here from your Amnio…... It's negative." "Does that mean the baby is ok?" "Yes, negative means everything is good. All your levels are fine." Sharon smiles and looks up at Todd as tears well up in her eyes, "It was normal. It's normal." Todd lets out a deep breath, "That's wonderful news. That's awesome Sharon." "Mrs. Kruder?" "Yes." "Would you like to know the sex of the child?" "Just a second doctor." Todd looks at Sharon, "What is it Sharon?" "The doctor wants to know if we like to know the sex? What do you think?" "Sure Sharon. Why not. You earned it for all that you've been through. Why not." "OK." Sharon places the phone back up to her face, "Doctor, my husband and I would like to know the sex of the baby." "It's a girl." Sharon drops the phone from her ear and looks back up at Todd standing next to her, "A girl. It's going to be a girl." Todd smiles from ear to ear, "That's why you're having a problem." Sharon looks puzzled, "What do you mean?" "Your body doesn't know how to handle a girl baby." Sharon smiles while she places the phone back up to her face. "Thank you doctor. Thank you."

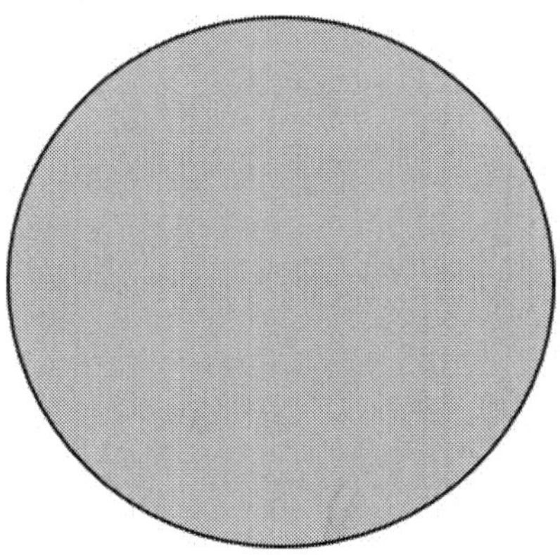

Seurat Dot Sixteen
USS SARATOGA

Nearing the end of Todd's first tour with the Squadron and soon after the birth of their daughter, Rebekah, Todd was assigned to the USS SARATOGA, an aircraft carrier that was conducting operations as part of a larger battle group presence in the Mediterranean.

Todd had been gone for several weeks. Sharon's primary means of communication with Todd was through "snail mail" or old fashioned letter writing. Computers were still not readily available and cell phone technology was still way off in the future. Sharon would write once a week. She would write Todd about what the kids were doing and how Rebekah was growing. Todd read Sharon's letters with great interest trying to respond in kind to each.

One letter that sticks out in Sharon's mind went something like this; "By the time you read this we'll be over the infestation of chickenpox so you won't have to worry. I've been trapped inside with the kids itching and being generally miserable…."

One afternoon, returning from the base commissary, Sharon had tuned the car radio to the Armed Forces Radio and Television Services (AFARTS) station. The news caster began the broadcast in the usual fashion, some banter, followed by the weather, and a look at world news. Sharon was shocked by what came next. The announcer begins with, "The aircraft carrier USS SARATOGA was involved in some sort of explosion with an unidentified NATO vessel operating in close proximity. First reports indicate that several crew members have been killed or injured. It's unclear at this point what sort of casualties may have occurred on the USS SARATOGA." A chill shoots down Sharon's spine. All Sharon knew was that Todd was on the ship. She had no easy way of communicating with him. Sharon drove back to the house, unbuckled the kids, and brought the groceries into the house. After placing a video in the VHS player for something the kids could watch she picked up the house phone and called a fellow spouse who she had become close friends with. "Hello" "This is Sharon, I was listening to the radio, coming back from the commissary, I heard something about an explosion and the SARATOGA. Do you think your husband can find out more?" The spouse on the other end of the phone knew Sharon was stressed, "Sharon, why don't you get the kids and come on over here. We'll get a hold my husband. Our kids can play together here." "That would be wonderful. I'll be over." "Good, I'll try to get a hold of my husband. I'll see you in a bit."

Sharon put the children back into the car and headed over to her friends. The children quickly ran off to play in the back yard as Sharon and her friend tried to get a hold of someone from the squadron for more word. After several attempts her husband calls back. "I'll find out what I can and give you a call right back. I'm sure he is fine. Don't worry." Sharon knew these words were meant to calm her nerves, but it wasn't working. Not knowing what exactly happened and where Todd was in all of it was wearing on her nerves.

Nearly an hour passes before the husband calls back. "Todd is fine. The explosion was on another ship not the SARATOGA. I don't know exactly what happened. I'm sure there will be an investigation but Todd is fine." Sharon let out a deep breath, feeling her nerves settle back to their "normal" state of having a spouse who is deployed.

Seurat Dot Seventeen
A Third Sac

Sharon and Todd's tour in Spain was coming to a close. They received their next set of orders. They would be moving to Monterey California so Todd could attend the Naval Post Graduate School. Their departure date was still about six months away. Plenty of time for several more deployments.

Sharon tells Todd one morning, "I think I may be pregnant." Todd looks back at Sharon, "What?" "You heard me. I made an appointment with the OB to get a pregnancy test." Their family now consisted of Joshua, Zachariah, and Rebekah. Sharon always wanted a larger sized family with an even number. Even though she had three children in quick succession she was excited about the idea of another child, another baby. Todd thought to himself, "I guess this could be it. We'll have our even number."

Sharon went back to the OB clinic to have a pregnancy test. The result was as she thought it would be, it was positive. She'd be having another baby although this time, in California.

The doctor at the base hospital ordered an ultrasound knowing Sharon would be PCS'ing back to the states. He wanted to ensure everything was fine.

Sharon entered the ultrasound room surprised to see the corpsman who she had known from previous visits in the pediatric clinic. Sharon laid back on the exam table, the technician placed the gel on her belly, and began to move the wand across her stomach. Sharon began wonder why it was talking longer than normal. "Why is it taking so long?" The corpsman replies, "I'm checking the third sack for another fetus." Sharon responds, "Not a funny joke to play on someone who has three little ones at home already." The corpsman looks at Sharon, "I'm not joking. Is there anyone you would like me to call?" Sharon took a deep breath, "Just keep doing what you're doing and we'll talk when you're done with the ultrasound."

The corpsman finishes the ultrasound, "The third sack is empty. It appears the fetus self-aborted...... But there are definitely two babies."

Sharon was in shock. She knew she was to be home soon but still had some errands to run and didn't want Todd to worry. She used a phone in the clinic and dialed the house number. "Hello?" Todd was expecting the duty officer and was surprised to hear Sharon's voice. "It's me, I just want to let you know that the ultrasound took a little longer than normal. I just didn't want you to worry." "Are you sure everything is all right? You sound a bit off?" "I'm fine, we can just talk when I get home." "Just tell me. Just tell me." Todd's mind immediately raced through a myriad of possibilities. Todd was instants so Sharon replied, "Well, are you sitting down?" "No, I'm standing why?" "You may want to sit down." "I'm fine Sharon, just tell me. What's wrong?" "Well like I said, nothing is wrong. At least I don't think it is. You know I was having an ultrasound today." "Yes." "Well, we're having TWINS." Todd hesitates replying.... "Twins? Are you sure?" Sharon responds, "Yes. In fact the technician saw three sacks but the third was empty." "Oh my God! Just come on home. Forget about running the errands."

Seurat Dot Eighteen
Flak Jackets

Todd was in his second squadron tour with VQ. This time the family moved to Whidbey Island to join up with VQ-1. The squadron recently completed a homeport change from Guam, completing the station move about eight months before they arrived.

The deployment schedule in VQ-1 was very similar to what they experienced in VQ-2. The main difference for Sharon was now she was in the states. Todd had completed a number of deployments when he was called up to the Executive Officer's office. The XO told Todd they needed to fill a critical billet in Riyadh, Saudi Arabia. A job needing to be filled in a matter of days. It was a staff position involving the assignment and flow of aircraft supporting the "no fly zones" over Iraq.

The news came as a surprise to Sharon. She learned to take everything in stride and seemed never to be shocked by what news Todd would bring home of an impending departure. She wasn't expecting this one though, possibly due to what the family was about to undertake.

When Sharon and Todd first arrived in Whidbey, Sharon had gone ahead, leaving Todd in Monterey to finish his Master's. Sharon wanted to be sure that Josh and Zach started school at the beginning of the school year in Whidbey.

She headed out weeks ahead of time to complete the function of "house hunting." A couple of days into her trip, Sharon stumbled on a rental. She learned quickly that the squadron's move to Whidbey caused a dramatic spike in housing demand on the island. There were two rental homes that had promise. One was larger than the other. The only problem, the smaller home took pets while the larger home did not. Their costs were nearly the same.

Sharon had to make a choice. Go with the larger home that didn't take pets or the smaller home that did. Sharon called Todd in Monterey and explained the options. After some discussion they both arrived at the same conclusion, "the dog will have to go."

After living in a 1400 square foot base house in Monterey where every inch of floor space was taken up with either furniture or kids toys, they both knew that space would be a welcome treat.

An added function along with the house hunting was the bonus of having to find schools for the five children. This effort often brought its own unique challenges. Sharon and Todd had to decide. "Put the kids in a public school?" Or put the kids in a "Private one."

This decision often required some investigative homework and even interviews with school staff. Sharon called back to Todd and discussed what she had learned about the local schools. The public schools were struggling, the feedback from parents was not glowing. Josh was heading into first grade and Zach into kindergarten. For Sharon these were crucial times when a child begins developing their base of knowledge and learning. As she talked with several parents in the local area she discovered a Christian school. Sharon went to the school, talked with the staff, and was very impressed by the learning environment they offered.

Sharon and Todd had just bought their first house after the lease on the rental was about to expire. Sharon had literally stumbled on a "For Sale By Owner" sign posted in front of a single story rambler. She pulled over and was able to get a quick tour inside. It wasn't as large as the rental but it wasn't as tiny as the base house in Monterey. She liked it. She liked it a lot. So much so that she called Todd at the squadron just after she returned home from the walk through. "You've got to see this house. It's wonderful. When do you think you can see it?"

Todd knew by Sharon's voice she was excited about the home, "I can come by today if that will work."

Buying a home was going to be a gamble. Sharon ran the personal finance numbers over and over again. Every penny was accounted for in the budget.

At one point Sharon mentioned to Todd, "Maybe my parents can help? I'll call my dad?"

Todd wasn't enamored with this idea. He didn't like the idea of being loaned money from family. They had to do this once already with Todd's father when they couldn't qualify for a car loan due to the fact that they moved too much.

Sharon and Todd made an offer on the house. The owners countered and of course Sharon countered that offer as well. The owners agreed to Sharon's price and we had a deal.

Sharon was surprised by Todd's news he would be leaving for Saudi Arabia in just a few days' time.

Sharon asked, "How long will you be gone for this time?"

Todd replied, "It could be up to three months, maybe less."

Sharon was wise in the ways of being a military spouse. She learned quickly that the Navy is pretty good about departure dates and not so good with return dates. What Sharon heard was, "I'm leaving in a few days and not sure when I'll be back."

"What about the move? Will you be here for the move?"

Todd replies, "We'll need to make some changes to the plan."

Their timeline was now significantly compressed. Sharon had gotten the owners of the house to allow Todd to store furniture in their garage ahead of the actual closing date. Todd piled furniture, mattresses, and boxes on top and in their red Jeep Cherokee. They shuttled load after load to the new house, completely filling the garage.

About three days after closing on the house and moving out of the rental Todd was off to Saudi Arabia. Sharon was left with cleaning the rental and stowing all the boxes from the move, while at the same time making friends with the new neighbors.

About six weeks into Todd's deployment Sharon was attending one of the children's soccer games. Sharon, standing next to a friend and fellow squadron mate of Todd's commented, all the while the children raced back and forth across the soccer field in front of her, "Oh yea. Did Todd tell you they were issued side arms?"

Sharon, shocked by the comment replies, "No. No he didn't."

The children continue to play their soccer game as he added, "Oh, don't worry. They issued them flak jackets as well."

This was more information than Sharon could process. Her vision was filled with lush green soccer fields, children running, and having a good time. It was difficult to comprehend such a dynamic. Difficult for Sharon to comprehend her husband could be in such a dangerous place.

News like this had to be managed. It had to be put away. If she allowed herself to reveal her true feelings Sharon knew the family stability she worked so hard to create would be affected. So, Sharon moved on, occupying her time with daily chores and the children activities.

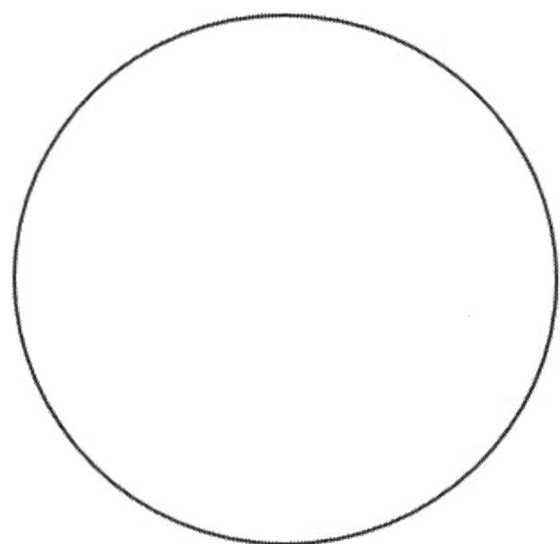

Seurat Dot Nineteen
Diapers and Baby Formula on the Doorstep

Another deployment meant another early morning departure. Starring at the clock positioned on the nightstand beside him, Todd reaches for the "off" button moments before the alarm would have gone off. Todd rolls over in bed, now facing Sharon, still drowsy from sleep. He kisses her and says, "I love you Sharon."

Sharon replies, "I love you too."

"Soon this will all be over."

Sharon responds, "I know. I know. Just one more. Right?"

"Yeah, just one more."

Todd gets up from bed as Sharon rubs her eyes clear of the morning sleep. Todd heads over to their walk-in closet and dresses with the door shut and only a sliver of closet light peering from under the door.

Dressed in his flight suite, gripping his green canvas gear bag in one hand while the other held his helmet bag he approaches Sharon now sitting up in bed preparing to start her morning.

Sharon knew that this early morning exchange of words was just that, words. She knew Todd had no control over the number of deployments. Sharon, like other spouses, looked at world news and events shown on the television differently from most. She wouldn't simply hear "Tragedy in the Middle East", or "Bombing Saudi Arabia". Sharon interpreted theses headlines as; "Your husband will not be coming home." Or, "Your husband will be leaving again soon, say goodbye once again." World News was just a prediction of another deployment or the extension of one already underway.

Todd walks into the living room and peers out the window into the darkened early morning sky. A flash of headlights momentarily lights up the living room as a car pulls up into the driveway.

"He's here Sharon."

"Ok, you be careful."

"I will. Say goodbye to the kids for me again."

"I will."

Todd wraps his arms around Sharon's waist, pulling her in close to his flight suite as he kisses Sharon one more time.

Several days go by without hearing from Todd, this was normal. Sharon's time was filled with activities revolving around the children. Extra challenging for any single parent in an area known predominately for rain and the phrase "sun breaks". Sun breaks, periodic moments of sun, a term familiar to many living in the Pacific North West.

The phone rings, "Hello?"

"Sharon, it's me."

"It's great to hear from you. How are you?"

"I'm fine. How are you and the kids?"

"Everyone is fine."

Todd was accustomed to this response just as Sharon was accustomed at saying it. It's not in Sharon's nature to complain or ask for help. She simply told Todd the facts. As long as Todd was gone, things on the home front would be fine, "There's nothing he could have done physically to help anyway. He was always thousands of miles away. But I could always count on him for moral support and advice. I knew at the end of the day, I had to handle it."

Todd was the senior member of the crew on this deployment. He was accustomed to reading faces and body language. He noticed one of the junior pilots was not himself.

Todd approached the pilot, "Hey, is there anything wrong?"

The pilot hesitated then said, "Yea. I just talked with my wife."

"Is everything ok?"

"Our baby has pneumonia and now my wife is sick as well. She doesn't have anyone to watch our toddler son."

"Would you be ok if I asked my wife Sharon to check up on her? Would that be ok?"

"That would be great. I think my wife would like that."

Todd called back to Sharon in Whidbey and explained the situation to her. Once Sharon heard the name she immediately knew the family was new to the squadron and the area. When Todd asked if she wouldn't mind checking up on her Sharon responded immediately, "Of course I will."

Todd gave Sharon her phone number and address. Sharon replied, "I'll give her a call and see what she needs."

"That would be great. I feel bad putting one more thing on your plate. I didn't know who else to call."

"Don't worry about it. I'd be more than happy to help, you know that."

"I know. I know you would be."

Sharon called the pilots wife and briefly spoke to her and determined what she could use. The pilot's wife was reluctant at first to accept help. She didn't want to inconvenience another spouse. Sharon insisted, "We're here to help each other. That's what we're here for. What can I do to help?"

The pilot's wife finally relented and mentioned a few things she could use from the commissary although she insisted Sharon just leave the groceries at the door step. She didn't want Sharon and the kids to become sick, she would have felt awful.

With the three older children in school for the day, Sharon gathered up the twins and headed off to the commissary where she picked up diapers, milk, and some cans of soup.

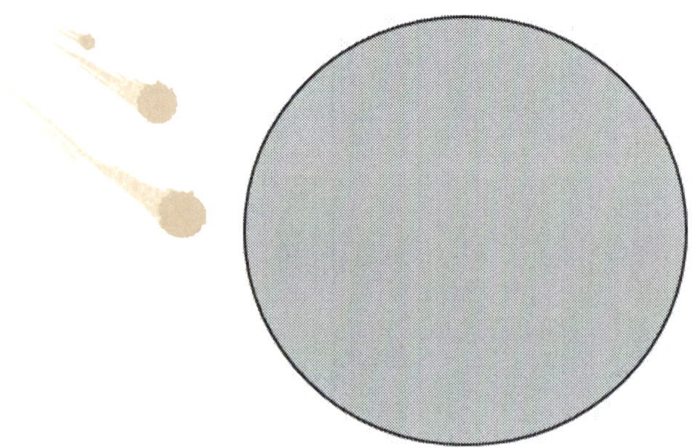

Seurat Dot Twenty
For Sale By Owner

Sharon and Todd had moved into their first home, taken out their first mortgage, and did it without needing a cent from family. There was a time that Todd thought he could stay in Whidbey. The thought made Sharon happy, a rare opportunity to stay in one place for more than three years. Over time, the possibilities began to look less promising.

The deployments kept coming. She had been single parenting for years. One evening, after dinner and the children were put to bed, Sharon looked at Todd, "I don't think I can do this anymore Todd."

Todd appeared puzzled, "Do what Sharon?"

"This. This life. Do you realize how many months you have been home this past year? Do you have any idea? Any idea at all?"

Todd paused before replying as he tried to think about Sharon's query, "I don't know. Why?"

"You've been home this year alone for a total of ten weeks. I'm talking a total of ten weeks, not even ten weeks straight. I'm TIRED OF SINGLE PARENTING."

"Wow, I didn't realize I had been gone that much. I'm sorry. I know you do a lot. I feel bad. Maybe I should get out. I've put in the time I owe. Maybe I should just get out."

"I hate to ask that of you. I know how much this is what you wanted. Is there anything else that you can do? Is there some other job you do in the Navy?"

Todd investigated a job change, a transition to the Aeronautical Engineering Duty Officer (AEDO) community, a restricted line designation. If accepted, Todd could continue to fly and meet his flight gates with fewer deployments.

One evening sitting around the kitchen table Todd discusses the possibilities of his transition to the AEDO community and what it would mean to Sharon and the family.

"I've looked into becoming an AEDO. They do acquisition and engineering. We'd keep our flight pay as long as I can get a flying billet."

"How do you do that?"

"I have to apply. They don't take many. It's tough to get into. I can try though."

"It sounds like it might be a good way to go. I can't see a down side."

"Well, there is one."

"What is it?"

"We'd have to move. We'd likely have to move to Patuxent River Maryland."

A look of disappointment comes over Sharon's face as she contemplates what Todd has just said. "We have only been in this house for a year. This was the first home we ever purchased. We bought this house thinking we'd be here for at least three years. Now I'm going to have to sell it?"

Sharon knew deep in her heart that if it meant they could be together as a family, the move would be worth it.

While at Nellis Air Force Base, Todd was told he was accepted into the AEDO community and would receive orders to Patuxent River Maryland. The good news was overshadowed as Todd returned home and was immediately told he would be heading out on another two month deployment.

The economy in the area was in a slump. Many who were leaving the squadron were forced to rent back their homes after failed attempts at selling them. The idea of renting back the home was frankly not an option they wanted to consider.

Todd was home long enough to scrub off the "for sale by owner" sign the previous owners had left in the corner of the garage and place the sign out in the front yard.

Sharon just cleaned up from lunch as the kids went to their rooms for some much needed "quiet time". Quiet time was Sharon's opportunity to recharge and relax, if only for an hour. Sharon had just sat down on the couch when the phone rings, "Hello?"

"Yes, I was just by your house. You are selling it correct?"

"Yes. Yes we are."

"Would it be terribly inconvenient if I were to stop by in an hour just to walk though it?"

Sharon paused thinking to herself, "How am I going to clean the entire house in enough time? What about my quiet time?"

Sharon replied, "Of course. That would be just fine."

"Wonderful. I'll be by in an hour. Thank you so much."

"No problem at all."

Sharon puts the vacuum away as the doorbell rings. Sharon opens the door to find an older woman standing just outside. The two exchange pleasantries and Sharon invites the woman into the house.

The buyer says, "Thank you so much for allowing me to see the house on such short notice. I drove by and saw the sign in the yard. The house looks wonderful from the outside. It's just what my husband and I are looking for. My husband is a retired Master Chief and loves this area. We're getting older and don't want a house with stairs. You know you can't find many ranch style homes?"

"Oh I know. My husband is in the Navy, I looked for some time before I found this house. Let me show you around."

Sharon gave the older woman a tour of the house and the entire back and front yard. Now standing at the front of the house the woman says, "You have a wonderful home. Thank you for showing me the house. I'll be in touch. Thank you again."

Two days later the woman she had shown the house to calls once again.

"Hello?"

"Yes, you showed me your home the other afternoon. I was wondering if my husband can see the house today."

Sharon replied, "Yes. That would be fine."

Sharon went over to the computer in the family room and started up the email program saying to herself, "Oh I hope you're able to check your email Todd. I hope you're not flying."

Sharon types out a note saying, "A couple wants to see the house again. What should I do?"

Todd was in Japan and happened to check his email. He read the note from Sharon and immediately picked the phone and dialed Sharon.

"Hello?"

"Sharon, it's me. I got your email. That's awesome news."

"I'm glad you think so. What do I do?"

"You show them the house. If they would like to make an offer let them. We can discuss it and get back to them. Let them know I'm deployed. I just can't believe that you have people looking at the house already. It's only been a few days. This is great."

Later that same day the couple arrive at the house. Sharon provides the couple the same tour she had done days before with the wife. The husband and wife begin to whisper to each other as Sharon leads them through the rooms. They head out to the backyard and then around to the front of the house.

The wife turns to Sharon, "We like the house. We like it a lot. How soon are you willing to sell?"

Sharon is shocked by the request, "I'm not sure what you mean. My husband doesn't PCS for about another six or seven months. We couldn't move out until then."

"Oh we understand. Would you consider selling the house and renting it from us?"

Sharon hadn't been thinking of renting back the house as an option, "I hadn't thought of that arrangement. I'd like to talk it over with my husband first. He's on a deployment but he can read email and he normally has time call me."

"That's just fine. How about we give you a call tonight with an offer. Talk it over with your husband and just let us know."

"That would be great."

That evening the couple called and made their offer. They offered the asking price of the house and an option to rent the house back. Sharon was excited and nervous all at the same time. The sign hadn't been in the yard for more than ten days, Todd was deployed, and she had offer that was the asking price.

Todd returned about two months later. The "For Sale By Owner" sign now no longer in the yard but propped up against a wall in the garage just as it had been before he left. In the time Todd was gone Sharon had single handedly sold the house, completed the closing, and entered into a rental agreement with the new owners.

Seurat Dot Twenty-One Talking Bear

Todd made it back from Iraq on leave, literally, just in time for the Holiday's. "Seeing him there in the airport terminal was JUST like a scene from a movie. I couldn't had gotten a BETTER Christmas gift!" The entire family was there at the airport to greet him.

Sharon and the kids were happily surprised to be pressed for time, "Todd had been able to change his flight plans when he landed in Atlanta. He was able to get a flight that would basically arrive at BWI in the amount of time it would have taken me to drive!"

Sharon and the kids arrived at the airport and rushed toward the terminal. "We entered at the lower level by baggage claim and I knew I had to get up to the second level. I had a choice to make, ether stay with the kids or race up the escalator steps and leave them behind me. I recall our daughter turning towards me as we rushed through the airport saying, 'Mom! Mom! Just GO! We'll catch up!' When I heard her say those words….. That's all I needed. That was all the affirmation I needed. I raced up the escalator steps leaving the kids to follow."

Sharon quickly made it to the top of the escalator and immediately began to scan the returning passengers, looking for someone, anyone, in a uniform as they passed by the opposite side of the security check point.

"It was super crowded. Because of Todd's height and build it would have been easy for me to miss him amongst all the people. I didn't have all the kids with me so I was worried he would miss me… I wouldn't have our normal posy surrounding me."

"I remember seeing Todd through the protective glass which separated the incoming passengers, still needing to go through security, and the returning passengers. I could see Todd walking behind that glass partition. I just couldn't get to him quick enough (in my own mind), there were so MANY people."

Todd turned the corner, now only about twenty yards away, no longer over four thousand miles, he was there with her, in the same time zone, in the same building, breathing the same air once again. "I couldn't hold back my excitement, I was as bubbly inside as a little child on Christmas morning. My Christmas gift had just arrived. As soon as I saw an opening I raced toward Todd and we engulfed each other in our open arms. I finally had him back, even if it was for just ten days."

Sharon and Todd were joined by their five children. The entire family wrapped their arms around each other, looking like a football huddle in the middle of the terminal, an obstacle of human beings oblivious to the crowds and noise around them. The excitement was electrifying. Everyone began to joke, laugh, and smile.

A decision was soon upon them. Should they assimilate themselves back into what was considered the norm or deviate from Kruder family tradition. For years, the family would spend time; preparing Christmas day dinner, make Christmas Cookies, watch *It's a Wonderful Life*, and attend midnight mass. This Christmas Eve was different, it was anything but the norm. This Christmas Eve called for a change, a deviation form tradition. Instead of heading home and carrying on with what was considered the tradition, the family agreed to simply head out to eat at a local Mexican restaurant. This may sound like a silly moment in time, however, for the family, it was the recognizing the time was different, it was recognizing this year wasn't like all the rest. "I had my husband back, the kids had their father back, back from war, and we agreed that the most important thing for us was just being together. I wanted to savor every moment. Every moment was precious. It was crazy, even though I was so excited to see Todd the moment was soon dampened by the sense it was short lived. Each precious moment I had him back was just a grain of sand falling into the bottom of the hour glass timer. I knew, in the back of my mind, the counter had already started. The counter that would count down to his inevitable departure, once again. His return to war.

"At the restaurant, we did something completely out of character for our family. We asked the waitress who was serving us to please take our picture. We had the kids huddle down at one end of the table as the waitress snap a photo. I wanted to capture the moment. I never told Todd this… Not until now that is. The real reason I wanted the picture was that I wasn't sure we would ever be together again. I wanted an artifact of that moment, forever in my memory. The photo sits atop our living room mantle even today."

"During Todd's ten days of leave, we didn't want to go anywhere really, we tried to keep things family centric. I never had ten days fly by so quickly."

The night before Todd was to leave Todd decided it would be nice to go out and eat, take a little burden off of Sharon. We loaded up the minivan and headed out for dinner. "I could feel this time wasn't anything like his return. The mood was somber, there was little joking, and even less smiling. The conversation felt forced. I knew it wasn't going to be the same…. I hadn't expected it to be this morose."

"The night before, our oldest son, Joshua, asked if he could drive us to the airport the next day. Todd thought it was a good idea, he knew how I loved driving expressways. I refused though. Not because I felt I couldn't use his help. I knew that this time, unlike all those departures in the past, I wasn't going to be able to hold myself together. I didn't want our son seeing me like that."

The next morning came quickly. Todd packed his small carryon bag and placed it in the back of the minivan and drove with Sharon back to BWI where he would catch another flight to Atlanta and then, eventually back to Iraq.

The conversation in the car was cordial and polite. "I knew Todd was doing his best to keep me from thinking about it. He did his usual bit trying to focus the conversation on the positive. He'd talk about happier times to come. As much as Todd tried to keep the moment upbeat I knew these last few hours would be it. I wouldn't see him again for another four or five months. He had come back into our lives to only once again to disappear."

Now at the airline counter, Todd received his boarding pass and asked the agent, "Pardon me Ma'am. Is there a way that my wife can go with me to the gate?"

"Oh yes. Certainly. I can print her a special pass. I just need to see a form of ID."

After providing the agent Sharon's ID we were handed another pass. This pass allowed Sharon to walk back to the gate for Todd's departure.

At the gate, there were a number soldiers wearing their camouflaged utilities. Many were listening to music or sat by the walls with their laptops watching a movie or simply surfing the web. "Todd and I sat across from the gate. It was dark in the terminal. He tried to talk with me, tell me the rest of the time would fly by. He'd tell me to think about the arrival. This departure was different from all the rest. In the past I knew he was flying high above the conflict, this time, he was on the ground, in the thick of it all."

The announcement came across the PA system. The gate agent announced the beginning of the boarding process. "Todd and I didn't move. We just sat there. He held my hand. I think he could tell I was more emotional than I had ever been. He stayed with me up until the last minute. We stood up from the chairs and hugged. I squeezed him tight in my arms, then we looked at each other, and kissed; our final kiss goodbye. I just wanted to freeze time. I knew he had to go. I knew I couldn't have my way. I just wanted him to stay home."

Todd approached the gate agent, handed the agent his ticket, and began to walk through the gate concourse. "I couldn't watch any longer. I didn't want him to see me in tears. I knew the tears were coming. As much as I tried to keep them in I knew I couldn't. I didn't want Todd's last image of me to be one of emotion."

"Little did I know that my decision to leave when I did meant I missed Todd's last wave goodbye. Todd had turned around just before disappearing into the concourse to wave at me…He couldn't find me because I wasn't there."

"I walked back to the car sniffling and wiping the tears from my eyes. I sat in the car and thought, 'I need to get myself under control, I have other responsibilities, I can't focus on my own emotions, I can't dwell on the negative, and I have to put my mask back on.'"

"I had gotten home. Talked with our oldest son Joshua. He was the only one home at the time. I told him I needed to go upstairs and do a few things. I knew I needed to pull myself together, everyone would be coming home from school. I told Josh I would be back down in a few minutes."

"I walked into our Master Bedroom and saw this little teddy bear wearing camouflage fatigues leaning against the center of my pillows. Todd always knew I like Teddy Bears. He bought one for me whenever he could while we were dating. We must have hundreds in the attic. I walked up to the bed and noticed one of the paws had a sticker which read, 'push me'".

While Todd was waiting to catch his flight from Kuwait to start his leave, he stopped in the local PX where he saw this "recordable Teddy Bear". Todd was reminded how much Sharon liked Teddy Bears. He could record a personal message for Sharon, "She could have my voice on this little bear and play back the words, 'I LOVE YOU' whenever she wanted. How cool would that be."

"I picked up the bear up off the bed and sat on our cedar chest. I began to press the paw pad with no results. I knew the bear must have a message recorded on it. I just couldn't get the message to play. It was frustrating. I knew that this little camouflaged Teddy Bear held something from Todd…. The bear represented my last connection with him. Something Todd had left behind to get me through the months ahead. I started to press on the bears paws with the same silent result. Sitting on the cedar chest, I realized I must have pushed the paw pads in a sequence which deleted the message. I was devastated. The experience brought a whole fresh set of tears. I couldn't believe I erased the message."

"Our daughter returned from her day at High School. She was unusually quiet and headed straight up to her room. I could her sniffling so I went into her room to see what was the matter." Rebekah looked at me. Her eyes red from crying. Mom, I was at school today and one of my girlfriends asked if dad had left again. I just started to cry. I don't know why. I just cried. This sucks."
"What could I tell her? I couldn't lie to her. I simply sat next to her on the bed, held her, and said, 'It does suck.'"

Seurat Dot Twenty-Two Car Bomb

The Morning started off like most of the others while Todd was deployed to Iraq. Sharon was the first to get up in the house of now four children. Josh, the oldest was away at college. Sharon conducted her typical morning routine which involved taking their two dogs out, getting the local newspaper and finally sitting down to have a cup of coffee.

One by one the children would make their way down the stairs. Some more awake then others. They would have a bowl of cereal, a pop tart, or a frozen chocolate chip waffle. Sharon would use this time to figure out where and what everyone was doing that day. Each had a sport, each had a place to be, it was Sharon's job to figure out how she could split herself amongst the kids so that each wouldn't feel slighted by the lack of her presence. It was important to Sharon she do this. It was important now more than ever. Sharon knew it meant more to her than to the kids to show support for what they were doing. Sharon believed she had to make up in some way for Todd's lack of presence. She had to be Mother and Father. She was the stability for what otherwise wise could have been a house of emotional hysteria and chaos.

Todd was in Iraq once again, after having spent about ten days of leave back at home around the holidays. Communications with Todd were minimal since he had left. Most communication was over email and a periodic phone call. Sharon and the kids knew generally where he was. She knew the name of the Forward Operating Base, FOB Warrior. She also knew he was in Kirkuk. A city in the Northern portion of the country. Beyond those simple facts, she knew little else about his location.

Rebekah, Nathaniel, and Ethan grabbed their lunches and headed out of the house for the bus stop. Zach started a bit later and worked right after school so he drove himself instead of taking the bus, a High School Senior privilege in the Kruder house.

Sharon had finished her first cup of coffee and turned the television on to catch a bit of the morning news. She had just enough time to catch about thirty minutes of the morning news. Zach fixed himself some breakfast as he told Sharon what his day was going to be like.

Zach placed his dishes in the dishwasher and joins Sharon in the family room for a few minutes as he finished getting ready to leave for the day. The television news personalities bantered between one another as was typical for a morning news program. The host suddenly stop their discussion and turn toward the world news reporter for some "breaking news." The newscaster states, "This just in from Iraq. A massive car bomb just occurred in the northern Iraq city of Kirkuk. We're told the explosion was massive reports of injuries to military personnel and the local population is still not known. We'll update everyone once we have more details. Back to you…"

Zach had just walked behind the couch Sharon was sitting on. Sharon's hands trembled as she heard the news, here nerves inside her became twisted as the newscaster said the words "Kirkuk" and "car bomb." Sharon was trying to process the news when Zach asks her, "Isn't that where dad is? Isn't dad in Kirkuk?"

Sharon was taken aback by his words. Never before have the children acted in such concern. Never before were they old enough to understand the consequences of what Todd was doing. Sharon knew, she always knew. She recalled the incident on the SARATOGA. She hoped to insulate the children from the harsh reality that could result. "Car Bombs, Explosions, Shootings had a whole new meaning in our house."

Sharon turned toward Zach and said the only thing that she could say, "Yes Zach. Dad's in Kirkuk." Sharon could tell that Zach was visibly concerned. "I'm sure he is fine Zach."

Zach responded, "How do you know for sure? Have you heard from him this morning?" The family knew that news from Iraq was always delayed.

Sharon looked at Zach, "I'll email your father and let you know when I hear back from him."

Sharon worked at the kids High School library. At the time her desk was situated in such a manner that she could see the students pass back and forth during class changes. Later that day while Sharon was working she had received an email from Todd, he was fine. A bit later, during a class change, Sharon looked up and saw Zach walking by. Zach looked into the library. Sharon looked back at Zach, raised her left hand high up into the air so he could see it, and made the simple gesture of a "thumbs up." Sharon knew the message was received. Zach nodded his head in receipt. No words were exchanged…. Just a simple gesture of a raised hand and a nod of the head.

Section Four
Living in the Fog of Depression

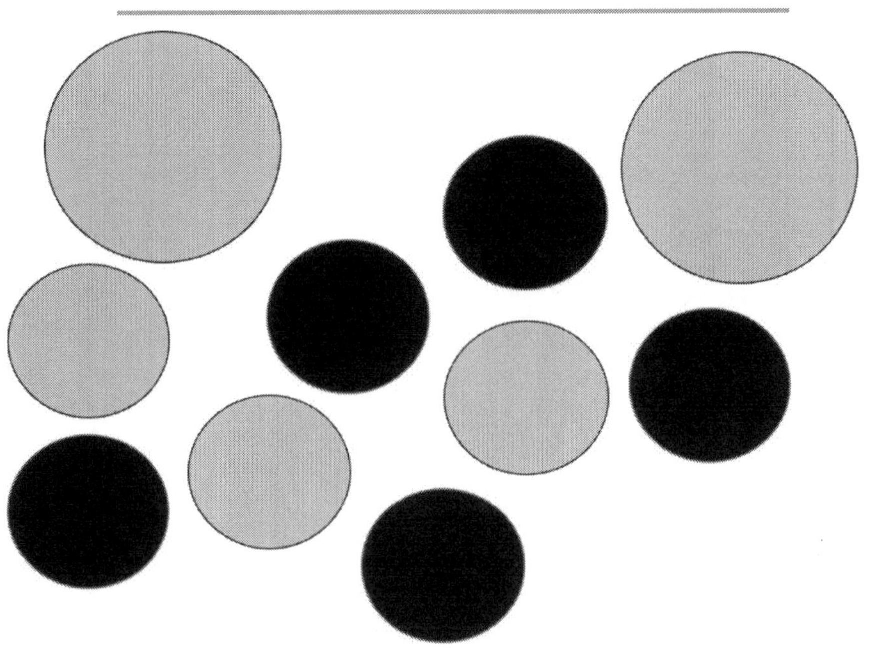

Seurat Dot Twenty-Three
Something Was Wrong

In the early days following Todd's return from his Iraq deployment Sharon felt things weren't the same. Sharon attributed it to the fact Todd was living in a war zone. "He wasn't use to our day-day living. He didn't see things the same way the family did. The only things that mattered to him were life and death. If it wasn't life or death, it didn't matter."

Sharon and Todd were married now for over twenty years. They endured numerous deployments and permanent change of station moves together. They weathered numerous emotional issues; Zach's tubes, the trip back to Bethesda during Sharon's pregnancy with Rebekah, bloodied noses, split lips, and broken arms. In Sharon's eyes, this was another exercise they had to deal with as a couple and as a family.

"Something happened to him, I noticed something about him had changed while he was still deployed. I felt that whatever it was would slowly go away. Things would come back to normal. Whatever it was wouldn't be permanent. I was willing to concede some of the changes to his behavior. I figured it wasn't permanent. He'd come back to me. I'd have the old Todd back."

The first morning of Todd's return Sharon joined him at the kitchen for a cup of coffee. Todd was standing by the kitchen island. Sharon comments to him, "You know. If you ever want to talk about what happened over there I'm here for you. I may not know what it was like but I'll be happy to listen." Sharon wanted Todd to know she was there for him.

Todd looked at Sharon considering his response, "I know Sharon. I'm fine." Those two words "I'm fine" were often used in the house to indicate, "I don't want to talk about it." Sharon could only imagine what Todd had gone through. She had no idea of what his day-day life was like. She hoped that Todd would open up to her, but she was wrong. Sharon could tell the experience had an impact on him.

Sharon could see that Todd was becoming visibly upset. Sharon figured it was way too soon. "Todd needed more time to process what he had been through. So I backed off."

"I could tell this was not the Todd I knew. There was something different. I could tell he was still trying to process what life was like in the house. The decisions in the house were not on the same scale as what he had to deal with when he was in Iraq. No one would get killed if we decided to have roast beef or chicken for dinner. An IED would not go off if we decided to go out to eat. These were not LIFE and DEATH decisions. His adrenalin did not have to be as keyed up. This is our life, and Todd was trying to figure out where his place was once again. He needed to find a new sense of purpose."

Todd tries to explain what it was like as his voice begins to crackle and his eyes well up with tears. He struggles to say the words that ramble through his head. Sharon pushes back on her kitchen chair across the hard wood floor, stands, and approaches Todd as he leans on the island. Sharon wraps her arms around his waist saying, "Its ok Todd. It's ok." In Sharon's mind she worried if it would ever be ok. It was just too soon to make that decision.

Sharon noticed Todd's eating habits had drastically changed. He had become very health conscious. Todd rationalized these changes as being "life style changes". He lost a lot of weight, dropping about thirty pounds in total. "Cake" was a four letter word.

Todd wanted to reintegrate into the family so he took some leave. During this time he took our daughter, Rebekah, to get her driver's license exam. He also volunteered to take the dogs for their annual checkup. While at the vet, Todd learned that one of the dogs was overweight. When he returned, he was obsessed with the idea. He mandated that we measure the food precisely. Only giving the dog the exact amount for her size. Ironically, Todd didn't want to exercise with the dogs. His answer was simply to curtail the dog's food.

During the first few weeks of Todd being home he was obsessed with eating healthy. There was no eating out. Interesting enough, Todd still needed to have cookies. "I was confused. Were we still allowed to eat deserts?"

Along with his obsession with food Todd exercised at least twice a day. He would jump rope for about 45 minutes, stopping every two minutes to do a minute of calisthenics then he resumed jumping rope. When he was done, his clothes appeared as though he had gotten back from the pool. They were drenched with sweat.

Despite his obsession with food and exercise he never, never, commented on anyone of the kids or my appearance. He never said to us we were overweight. He simply wanted all of us to eat healthier.

The command Todd was assigned to conducted a periodic welcoming back of the IA's, a sort of, town hall home coming. Todd RSVP'd although the date of the event changed from what was originally planned. The date slipped to the right and now fell on top of Zach's graduation from High School. "I wanted to keep things the way they were supposed to be. I wanted to take Zach out for dinner after his graduation. Doing so meant we couldn't make the beginning of the ceremony. Todd wouldn't have it. He had to be there at the beginning or there was no point in going at all. We didn't attend the home coming and I felt badly. I was afraid Todd felt I was blowing off the importance of his deployment. I chose Zach over Kirkuk. That pissed Todd off."

Seurat Dot Twenty-Four
Outer Banks

Sharon and Todd exchanged ideas about plans for his return from Iraq. Sharon learned Todd didn't want to be around crowds of people when he returned. This caused Sharon to consider what options might be available.

One afternoon, while Sharon was at work, she struck up a conversation with one of the High Schools front office secretaries. Sharon explained the situation and the Secretary replied, "Every year my family and I get together in the Outer Banks. We rent a house by the water, it's a great time, very relaxing."

Sharon listened with great interest. They had never done anything like that before. In the past, family vacations were tightly budgeted, often conducted in the local area to avoid the cost of a hotel.

Sharon came home from work that day and began to search on house rentals in the Outer Banks. She looked at several rental management sites. She typed in her requirements such as, pool, close to ocean, Wi-Fi, and four plus bedrooms. Several houses began to look promising. Now she just had to see if they were available for the dates she wanted. Her calendar requirement siphoned off a few more houses leaving just a couple to choose between. Everything looked doable, now she just need to see what Todd thought of the idea.

The phone rang in the late evening, Sharon new it was Todd. He tried to call near the same time so that Sharon could be available. Their phone calls consisted of mostly updates on the kids; the latest on scholarship applications, and the high school sports scores.

Sharon introduces a new topic, "How would you feel about renting a house in the Outer Banks. I talked with one of the front office secretaries and she couldn't say enough about it. It sounds like it would be very relaxing. What do you think?"

Todd paused briefly as he contemplated the possibilities, "Well it beats going to someplace where there'd be a lot of people. I really don't want that. How much is it though?"

Sharon knew that this could be the deal breaker. After years of raising five children and living on Todd's salary alone Sharon and Todd became very frugal. Sharon chose her words carefully, "It's not bad really. We'd be going before the 4th of July."

Sharon went on to describe the house and its amenities. Sharon waited for his reply. "Sure, what the hell. Let's just do it. Who would be going?"

Sharon knew that was a good question, she assumed everyone. Josh their oldest was working between semesters in college. Like all the Kruder kids he was required to pay his own way. Josh worked during the year on campus and was fortunate to have a paid internship. Zach, similarly to Josh, had to pay for college. He too needed to work during the summer. This left Rebekah, Nathaniel, and Ethan.

Sharon replied, "Well, I would say it would be the three younger ones for sure. I don't know if Josh or Zach can go though. You know they both have to work."

Todd replies, "Yea. I wouldn't want to impact their work. I know they need the money. Besides, this is just for a week."

Sharon knew this was a time for family to be together, she also knew how important it was for the children to understand commitment, financial independence, and a strong work ethic. Sharon and Todd weren't ready to sacrifice those ideals, not for a week vacation anyway. Sharon and Todd left the decision up to them to decide. Although due to their upbringing and way of thinking, they opted not to go, and work instead.

Sharon hoped that the vacation would be just what Todd and the family needed. A time to simply relax. Relax in a large house, relax in the pool, and relax on the beaches. Just relax and re-acclimate.

Josh and Zach remained behind as the rest of the family packed the car and headed out on their five hour drive to the Outer Banks. Sharon had taken care of every detail. As they approached the Outer Banks the traffic worsened with a new wave of renters all converging on the location at the same time. Sharon could see Todd was becoming anxious and impatient with the bumper to bumper traffic.

Arriving at the rental management office Sharon went into the building and came back out with the keys and paperwork. They drove from the management office to the rental house. The house was beautiful. A three story wood framed home with five or six bedrooms in all. A wooden deck off each of the three floors all connected by a set of wooden stairs, a built in pool, a hot tub on second floor deck, and only a few minutes' walk to the beach. The sounds of the surf could be easily heard from the house. It's everything Sharon had hoped it would be, and then some.

Sharon noticed a fidgetiness in Todd's demeanor. He was visibly uneasy. Sharon asked him, "Is there something the matter?"

Todd replied, "I'm fine. I think I just need to work out." Sharon knew it was a bit odd for him to make such a request, especially when the idea was to relax. Sharon knew Todd had to do something though so she silently agreed.

Sharon watched as Todd changed into his workout gear, grabbed a jump rope, and headed to the outside of the house. He moved some deck furniture and began to jump rope. He would stop, do some calisthenics, then jump rope again, do some calisthenics, jump rope again. He'd do this for an hour or more. He'd do pushups on the concrete, he'd do sit-ups on the concrete. "He looked like a mad man at times. It was just too intense. He just loved the fact he was engulfed in sweat. I was very worried about him."

One of the days the rains came. Sharon, Todd, and the children were now held captive by the weather in the house. Todd's nervousness became more and more apparent. He tells Sharon, "I need to work out."

Sharon looks at Todd saying, "What? You know it's raining out. It's lightening and thundering as well. I don't think it's a good idea?"

But, Todd was determined, he changed into his gym shorts and shirt. He headed down to the lower level bedroom. He walked into one of the bedrooms, moved the furniture so that an open space was available on the floor. He started some calisthenics, then Sharon hears something odd. Sharon begins to hear a pounding on the stairs. The pounding becomes louder, and louder. Sharon puts a book down that she had picked up to read as she sees Todd racing up the three flight of stairs. Todd quickly turns around and races back down to the first level. He repeats this activity for about two minutes before going back into the bedroom for more calisthenics.

During this time our daughter Rebekah asked her mother, "How about we go out to the store?"

Sharon replied, "No. No. I'm good." What Sharon was really thinking was, "I can't leave your father like this. I'm afraid he will hurt himself if we leave him alone. I can't leave him."

Sharon wasn't sure what to make of this activity. She felt it was simply a way for Todd to use some his pent up energy. She knew something more was wrong though when Todd would go off, change, and do this again, and again. Sometime two or three times a day while on vacation.

Sharon realized that the week away didn't accomplish what she had hoped it would have. She wanted the two of them to relax. Instead, Todd seemed even more nervous and fidgety. It was as if he couldn't relax. Down time for him was like a demon to him. Sharon also realized that a change in the environment alone wasn't enough. Todd's problem wasn't solved by simply changing his surroundings. The time in the Outer Banks only made Sharon more concerned for Todd's wellbeing. At that moment Sharon realized the six weeks since Todd had been home were not enough for Todd to re-acclimate, it was going to take longer, just how long was the question. A question Sharon did not have the answers to.

Seurat Dot Twenty-Five When A Spouse Needs Help

Sharon was an avid reader her entire life. It was not uncommon for Sharon to have checked out multiple books from the Public Library all at the same time. The living room book shelves were stocked with novels that she had read, some she had even read twice. It was natural for Sharon to turn towards books for advice on the subject of returning military and the impact on their families.

Sharon had gone to the public library and checked out several books. She paged through each book with great interest in hopes of finding the one thing that may lead to some answers. "I knew there was something wrong. I wanted to know if there was something I could do to have him express his true feelings. I felt if could just get him to talk to me and share his experiences it would help. He didn't want anything to do with the subject. He was closing off a section of his life to me and I couldn't figure out why. There was something more he wasn't sharing."

One afternoon Todd noticed the title of one of the books Sharon was reading. It contained the words PTSD. Seeing this, Todd grew very angry, and became defensive yelling, "Why are you reading that crap? I don't have PTSD. I'm fine. I told you that before. Don't waste your time reading that crap."

"I felt the books could hold an answer. They could give me questions I could ask. Maybe there was a study or finding as a result of a study. The books might give me some options that I didn't know existed. From this point on I continued to read the books, I just simply didn't read them when he was home or around. I placed them out of his sight and in a basket beneath the coffee table, out of his sight."

One afternoon on a weekend when Todd exploded with a rant of, "There's nothing wrong with me. Did you ever think it could be you who has the problem?"

"Todd's words actually made me doubt myself. Maybe I was demanding too much. Maybe it was me. I held his opinion in high regard. What reason did I have to stop?"

"I didn't know where to turn. I wasn't getting the answers I needed from the books I was reading. I wanted a solution, nothing the books offered were working. I needed a way to deal with the arguments we were having. I knew the constant arguing was having an impact on the kids. During this time Todd tried to deny there was a problem and I tried to research the problem. There was no us. We were in a blame game with each other. We weren't working together towards a solution."

Sharon knew she needed to get help herself. Todd's depression was now engulfing her and the kids. If Todd wasn't going to get help, she was. Sharon knew that if Todd caught wind of her seeking treatment he would get upset, she didn't want that. Sharon resorted to something that she never had to do in the twenty plus years she had been married to Todd. She turned to lying. Sharon formulated a cover story. She told Todd that she was going to weight watcher meetings in the evening once a week. Todd bought it. He was oblivious to what Sharon was actually doing.

Sharon arrived one evening for her first talk therapy session. Sharon introduced herself to the women as they both sat down. The therapist wanted to open the session with a prayer. She asked Sharon if she was ok with it. Sharon wasn't expecting the request and felt it was just easier if she simply complied. The therapist reached out toward Sharon's hands, grasping them as she led the two in a short prayer. Sharon was uncomfortable with this approach. Sharon wanted to talk to someone who could help her understand what she was going through and ways she could use to fix what was broken.

During this time, Todd received news he had made the rank of Captain. Along with the promotion came another set of orders. This time his orders would take him to Norfolk. The conversation that Sharon and Todd had over moving to Norfolk was a difficult one, "No, we're not moving. If you go, you go alone."

"I didn't want Todd to take these orders. I thought I had done enough with my duty when he went to Iraq. Once again, I'm being asked to disrupt my life. It was easier if I just stayed in the house and left the kids in school. Todd didn't seem to be bothered by this fact. It was almost a 'too bad too sad' sense I received from him." So, for the first time in their military life, they would not be going together as a family. He would be going it alone, a "geo bachelor".

"With the knowledge of Todd being in Norfolk during the week, the kids in school, and my full time job, I knew there wasn't going to be enough time to continue the sessions. So I stopped after about six weeks."

Seurat Dot Twenty-Six
Sunday Departures

Todd did the four and a half hour drive every Sunday down to Norfolk. He departed between 4:30 or 5:00 in the evening, after an early dinner, in order to miss the 9:00 P.M. tunnel lane closure. He returned home each Friday night after stopping by the Commissary to pick up groceries. Most of the time he would be home around 7:00 or 7:30 in the evening. Todd had made a promise to Sharon when he received the orders, "I'll be home every weekend." He was true to his word.

"We were cordial enough with each other when Todd got home. Todd just isolated himself from everyone. It wouldn't be long before the 'non communication' would start. Normally we'd make it to Saturday morning before something would set Todd off. It didn't have to be much it seemed."

By the time Saturday morning rolled around the conversation was limited. "I tried to talk about what was going on and he just didn't seem to care. It was almost like he was happier when he was away. His emails to me during the week could make me smile. It was like he was a different person when he was in Norfolk."

Every now and again the quiet of the morning would erupt in an argument. "He would get so frustrated and agitated with me it seemed. I couldn't do anything that would make him happy. I'd often cry out of pure frustration. That didn't even seem to affect him."

"I couldn't wait for Sunday to arrive and for Todd to leave. It had gotten that bad in the house. The house didn't feel like a home when he was there. It had a dark and miserable feeling to it when he was there. I couldn't wait for him to leave to have the house return to normal."

"With our kids heading into college and with all their activities during the week, I had more than enough to deal with. I just didn't have the drive within me to placate him simply because he came home for a day and a half. I knew the house was working the way it was. Todd was gone all week and when he was home he wasn't really even here. He would do his laundry, get some food for the week, and workout. It was as if we were just a stop off."

"When Todd left for all those deployments in the past I remember feeling terrible inside, I didn't want him to go. I wanted nothing more than to have him show back up at the front door saying, 'They found someone else to go.' That of course never happened. So when I looked forward to seeing him go I knew something was terribly wrong."

"The mood in the house changed after Todd left on Sunday's. The children talked to me and we laughed. The house became warm again, to some degree even more relaxed."

One Saturday morning, Sharon became frustrated with Todd's lack of communication. Sharon became so frustrated she contemplated telling Todd the truth about her past therapist visits. She knew Todd would be upset. She knew she had never lied before, not like this. What other recourse did she have? Sharon began to think, "I should tell him what I'm doing. Maybe he'll see there is a problem. It's not just me. I want to help us. I want to help us get back on track." Sharon realized telling Todd about the therapist visits was a risk, a risk that could back fire, and push Todd even further away.

Sharon decided it was her only opportunity to make a difference. She decided to tell Todd. "I've tried to figure out what is wrong with us and I have no answers. I've seen a therapist. I haven't been going to weight watchers like I said I was. All those times you thought I was at a weight watchers meeting I was really seeing a therapist."

"You've what? Are you kidding me? Why?"

"There's something wrong between us. I just want the old Todd back."

"I've told you I don't have a problem. I just can't believe you lied to me. Why didn't you just tell me?"

"I would have but I know how you would react. I needed to talk to someone. You don't talk to me anymore. You don't say a word to me half the time. You come down the stairs, have your coffee, and read the paper. You don't even acknowledge me. You just do your laundry and exercise."

Little did Sharon know when Todd left for Norfolk that Sunday afternoon he could not forget what Sharon told him. He could not forget the fact he was so immersed in the fog of his own depression he neglected to see what was happening to his wife and family. They had been sucked into his fog. Todd struggled with acknowledging his illness. He knew deep down inside he wasn't right, Something was wrong. Sharon's actions were just another sign. The books should have been a sign. The attempts by Sharon to talk about his problems should have been a sign. These were Todd's "ships bell" ringing in the fog, warning Todd of the collision course he was on, a collision course with the ultimate in Self-Harm, suicide.

Todd arrived in Norfolk that Sunday evening around 9:00. He carried his bags up to his fifth floor room. He placed his bags down by his side, walked up to the steel railing that looked out onto the base. He gripped the railing with both hands. Leaned forward at his waist and contemplated his death. He pushed his wife to the brink. He'd done untold emotional damage to his children. He was by his own accounts, a failure. He had come back from Iraq, not a hero, but a failure. He left the soldiers behind.

Todd told his therapist months later when asked why he didn't do it, commit suicide that night. Todd replied, "I was chicken. I was a coward."

When Todd awoke the next morning he knew something had to be done. He had to get help. In the long run, Sharon's tactic worked. It drove home to Todd the realization his depression, his illness, was affecting not only himself but others around him.

Seurat Dot Twenty-Seven
Raking Leaves

"Todd didn't care about anything anymore. He use to touch up paint the walls when they would get dirty from scuff marks or hand prints. He didn't anymore. He use to take care of the yard. He simply made one of the kids do it now. He didn't seem to care about anything or anyone."

"I mentioned to Todd how the lawn needed to be raked. I'm sure that comment just resulted in another argument." One Friday night, when Todd returned from Norfolk and groceries he headed up the stairs to get changed. When he came back down to the kitchen Sharon asked, "Where are you going?"

Todd put his jacket on and replied, "I'm heading outside for a bit to rake up some leaves."

Sharon notices how dark it was getting, "It's going to be dark soon. It's too late to rake leaves?"

Todd puts his hand on the doorknob to the garage door, "It's fine. You wanted the leaves raked didn't you?"

Sharon realizes Todd had made up his mind, "Yea, but I didn't mean for you to do it on a night when you just got home."

"I've got the time now." Todd opens the garage door and heads into their shed to find a rake.

Todd starts to rake the front yard. The star's begin to shimmer in the cold night sky above. Todd was raking for about thirty minutes when one by one he is joined by his family. Todd remained obsessed with raking despite the darkness and the cold that began to take hold.

Todd places the rake onto the ground and walks into the house appearing moments later with the keys to his jeep in his hand. He walks around to the driver side door, starts the engine, and repositions the car so the beam of the headlights appear across the front yard.

Todd continues to rake. Sharon later asks, "I think this is good enough Todd. I think this is good for now."

Todd looks over at Sharon, "You can go in if you want. I got this. I want to finish." Todd looks back down at the leaves and continues to rake.

Todd stayed outside that evening for about three hours, raking the leaves by the headlights of the jeep. He raked until he finished. Just as he said he would.

"I just knew it was best to go along with what he wanted. I f I were to force the issue I'm certain he would have exploded and gotten angry. The kids and I didn't need that. Besides, I knew he would be heading back to work Sunday evening. Work was a place he seemed to find some happiness."

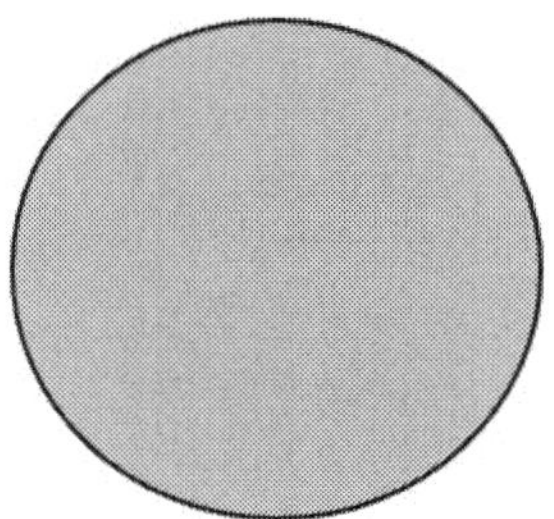

Seurat Dot Twenty-Eight
Effects of Therapy

"I was very surprised when I received an email from Todd saying he had an appointment with a therapist and that he had seen the local flight surgeon. I was hoping this would be it. This would make things better. This could be the answer I was looking for. I knew this wasn't in line with the typical military character. He was finally putting himself out there. It was a risk for him and I knew it."

The effects of his help was nearly immediate. The most immediate effect was on our ability to communicate with one another. "The simple fact that he was seeking help gave me hope."

After about two weeks of being on Zoloft and seeing a therapist I noticed traits of the husband who I knew and loved. Todd was less irritable and abrupt. "I felt this was going to be the answer. We had found a solution. This was going to work for us."

Todd was in a therapeutic plan for several months before he discovered during an annual flight physical he was no longer qualified. He had to be off all therapies for six months. He also learned that not being qualified meant his flight pay would stop.

"When I learned about these changes I told Todd his health was more important than the qualification and the money. We would adapt."

"Money was more important to Todd. I could see it in his eyes. I could tell he wanted me to agree with him. He wanted me to agree that money and the distinction of being a Naval Aviator was more important. I couldn't and I wouldn't."

It wasn't long after Todd's flight physical that he stopped his medication and talk therapy sessions. "Todd didn't tell me he was stopping his therapy. Only after I asked him how it was going did he mention to me he stopped."

His denial took over once again, this time flamed by the stigma associated with mental health. Todd believed he was now cured, only having been on medication for several months. "Todd was far from cured. We were working on things, making improvements, we were communicating more.... All if it was getting thrown out the window. I was concerned where we would go from here. How our home life would be affected? Our marriage? I knew how bad it could get and didn't want that again. Work was the only thing that kept Todd happy."

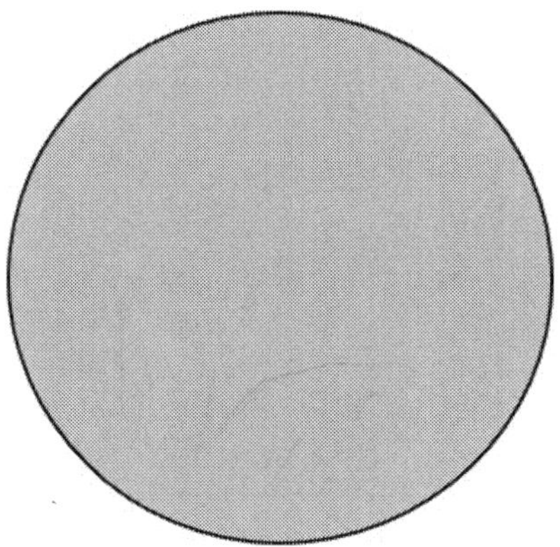

Seurat Dot Twenty-Nine
Another Set Of Orders

Now at Norfolk for a little over a year, Todd knew the Norfolk orders were not long term. Before issuing the orders, the detailer told Todd, "These are going to be written for two years but as soon as we can, we'll get you back up to Patuxent River." A little over a year went by when the detailer sent Todd an email indicating they have a replacement in mind.

Todd mentioned the email to Sharon, "They may have found a replacement for me here. I could be coming back to Pax." Sharon acknowledged the fact, but deep inside felt Todd wasn't ready to give up the job, "He seemed happier there then when he was at home."

Sharon and Todd had been through a lot since he took the orders to Norfolk. Their marriage nearly crumbled and Todd's depression led him to seriously consider suicide. Todd sought treatment for the first time, but also felt the pain of the stigma, and withdrew himself from his therapy, convincing himself and mothers he was now fine.

Todd heard about a job working as the Executive Assistant to the Admiral who oversees all of NAVAIR. This was not like the other jobs Todd had taken in the past, this one required Todd to be personally interviewed by the Admiral. Todd described the duties of the job to Sharon. "I could tell Todd was excited about the prospects." What Sharon really thought was, "What's the point of you coming home? It sounds like all you're going to do is sleep in the bed at night...."

There were about a half dozen of candidates for the job in total and Todd was just one. Todd returned home feeling less than confident about the interview. He didn't feel he had a chance at the job. Sharon had mixed feelings, "On one hand, I knew the job would make him happy. On the other hand, I knew he would be so busy that the kids and I would never see him."

Todd arrived home one Friday afternoon and was ecstatic. On the drive home he had received a phone call from the Admiral himself telling Todd the job was his if he wanted it. Todd had already accepted. The news was met with mixed emotions by Sharon, "I had to wrap my brain around the fact that Todd would be living at the house but gone most of the day."

Todd began the new job in late November. "Todd's work day were unbelievable, he would get up around 4:00 in the morning and return around 8:00 or 9:00 in the evening. I would save him something from dinner, he would eat whatever was left, and be in bed by 9:00 in the evening or as soon as he finished. He would come home tired and exhausted and not want to talk about his day. It was like this every day, Monday through Friday. The weekends were spent on his blackberry. Todd would say he wanted to spend time with me on the weekends. We would go to the commissary together although Todd spent the entire time on his blackberry, typing emails or talking to various people. If he wasn't on the blackberry he was catching up on his sleep. It was this way there and back. At the house, if Todd wasn't doing work, he was working out. He spent very little time with the family."

Sharon got tired of asking Todd for help, "Todd's physical body was here in the house but he had no interaction with us. I couldn't rely on him to do anything. It was a reuse." I knew from reading various things online that the EA job would be busy. I was floored that he wanted a job like Norfolk and this one. Where did the family rank in Todd's priority? It seemed like whatever made him happy is what he did. Family wasn't on his priority list." For Sharon, this was akin to Whidbey, when Sharon told Todd that she didn't want to do this alone anymore; "there was no more us."

"In some ways this job was even worse than Norfolk. He was here physically but he was always mentally at work."

Unbeknownst to Sharon, Todd was nearing his breaking point once again. Their marriage nearly nonexistent, constant fighting, and Todd pushing everyone out of his life, he once again seriously considered suicide, this time with sleeping pills prescribed by a doctor after he returned from Iraq. His attempt interrupted by his youngest son, he decided to get help once more. Todd contacted the local flight surgeon, explained what had happened in Norfolk, and attempted to convince the doctor it was "marital problems" and not depression. By doing so, Todd had hoped to avoid being labeled as depressed. A label he knew would mean loss of flight status and flight pay. Todd was placed back on Zoloft and referred to the behavioral health clinic on base. After one appointment he had convinced the therapist his problems were "marital". The doctor agreed to see Sharon and Todd in a couple's therapy type session. Sharon attended two or three of these sessions with Todd.

"I saw Todd trying to get help and I didn't care that Todd was blaming our marriage on the problem. I guess I hoped the therapist would see there was something more going on. It was more than marital problems."

Once again Todd has a conversation with the Flight Surgeon who reiterated the fact that he could not be on medication and in therapy and still keep his flight status and flight pay even if it were marital related. The loss of both was still too much for him to bare. After only several weeks of being on Zoloft and about five visits to the therapist he stopped, falling victim to the stigma of depression yet again.

After Todd stopped his medication and therapy for the second time Sharon noticed Todd was reaching for over the counter mental health remedies Sharon knew Todd wasn't fine and still in need of help, "Looking back on it now it's clear to me Todd needed to stay in a therapy. He still needed help."

Sharon knew she had to tread cautiously, Todd's career was the only thing keeping him going. It was the only thing keeping him happy. If she called the doctor or therapist behind his back she could end his career. "Up to now, I never knew Todd was suicidal. I never knew it had gotten that bad."

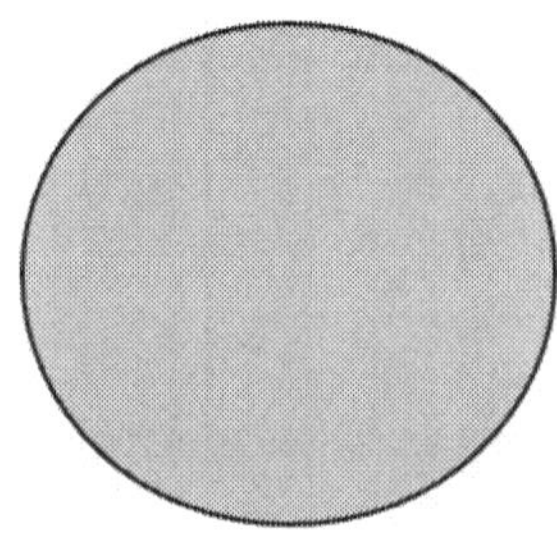

Seurat Dot Thirty
Break-In

While performing the duties as the Admiral's EA, Todd arrived home around 5:30 in the evening, several hours earlier than normal. He parked the car just outside the garage which was normal given the unusual demands of the job.

Sharon, surprised by the garage opening and not expecting Todd for some time asks him as he walks into the house, "Why are you home so early?" Although one look at him gave it away. Sharon could tell he wasn't feeling well. His face was pale and his body appeared stiff.

Todd mumbled his response, "I don't feel well, I'm just going up to bed."

Sharon thought it was exhaustion that made him feel the way he did, "I figured he just needed some rest. Not that one night would do anything…. It was better than nothing."

Even though he was tired and didn't feel well he dutifully gathered up his things for the next day and prepositioned them in the car, just as he would do every night after returning from a day at work.

Todd's alarm went off at the usual 4:00 in the morning. Sharon rolled over to her side waiting to hear the usual sounds, front door closing, the lock being turned, the car door opening, the door closing, the engine starting, and the engine noise fading as Todd drives down the driveway. Knowing that an hour later her own day would begin.

Sharon checked off each sound in her head, the front door, the car door…… Todd opened the driver's side door opening and closing. Only this time, she thought something was wrong. The engine didn't startup. Instead, she hears the driver side door open and close once again soon followed by the opening of the front door to the house, "I assumed had forgotten something."

What Sharon didn't know had happened….. Todd sat in the car, closed the driver's side door and reached for his iPod, "Where is it. Here's the cable, it's plugged in, maybe it fell to the floor?" Todd reached down to the passenger side of the car and began to feel around the carpet. "What's going on? Where is my iPod?" Then it struck him, "Did someone break into the car? No." He then recalled, "My wallet. I left my wallet in the car.

Son of a bitch!" Todd flipped the glove box open and placed his hand into the deep box. His hands fishing in the darkness. "My wallet! There it is!" He plucked the wallet from the depths of the glove box, flipped on the map light, and peered into the contents. Todd first looked for his credit cards and military ID. "There all there." Then he opened the wallet to check for the money, "Son of a bitch! They took my cash. Those bastards!" Todd was fuming with anger. His iPod taken, his money gone. "The candle, did they take the candle?" He reached back into the depths of the glove box and felt inside once again. His fingers probing from one corner to the other. "They even took the god damn candle!" Todd was now even more pissed.

Sharon hears the door slam shut and moments later Todd was standing by her bedside, standing there in disbelief that someone had broken into his car. Sharon asks, "Todd, what's wrong?" "Someone stole my iPod and all my cash."

"What?"

"Someone stole my iPod and cash."

"Wasn't your car locked?"

Todd paused as he carefully considered his reply. He started to think back to the evening before, when he came home early not feeling well; "Shit! Son of a bitch! I mustn't have!"

"What? You didn't lock your car?"

"No! I must have forgotten to lock it. I can't believe someone would have broken into my car. It was sitting just outside the house."

"Did they take anything else? What about your credit cards?"

"No. There's still here along with my drivers license and military ID."

Sharon is thinking, "The cards may be compromised already. I'll need to stop the credit cards."

"We need to call the police and report it. I'm late for work."

Todd stormed out of the bedroom and went to work. "He didn't even consider the fact that the robbery could have been in progress, or that the people who did this were still lurking outside around the house."

Sharon got up from bed and headed down to the kitchen. Sharon called the police first and was told it would take about twenty minutes since it wasn't considered an emergency. Sharon then called the credit card companies and reported the cards compromised.

During this time our oldest daughter comes down to the kitchen as the front door doorbell rings, it was the State Police. Sharon invited the officer into the house. Sharon, the officer, and our daughter sat at the kitchen table as Sharon relayed the details of the incident for the police report. The officer asks, "Is the car in question in the driveway?"

Sharon replied, "No. My husband took it and left for work."

Mildly surprised, the police officer said, "There isn't much they can do except take a report."

Sharon responded, "That's fine. I just didn't want it to go undocumented. In case other's in the neighborhood should be affected."

The police officer finished taking down the notes on the report and left the house. Our daughter asks, "Would you like me to stay home this morning?" She could tell that you were visibly upset over the ordeal.

Sharon answered, "No, thanks for the offer but I'll be fine."

It was this moment when Sharon TRULY realized it was just her. Just her and the kids. There was NO us. No husband.... I had to take care of everything. It simply brought it to the forefront just how alone I really was."

"It wasn't that I feared for my safety. It was just me and me alone to fix it. It really hurt."

Seurat Dot Thirty-One
Self-Harm

After about fifteen months as the Admiral's EA Todd was up for another set of orders. Todd looked at various opportunities outside of NAVAIR and away from Patuxent River Maryland. During his tour with the Admiral Todd had applied for numerous Major Program Manager Positions within all of DoD. At one time, he even interviewed for a position at SPAWAR San Diego. "He seemed frustrated. Frustrated that he couldn't find a job that would be as challenging as the EA job, as the Norfolk one, and even as his Iraq tour."

"I was thrilled that Todd seemed to finally recognize the fact I wasn't going to move again. It forced him to look local. Since Iraq, he was never here. He could finally get some down time. It was going to be a plus, a good thing in my eyes. He could finally relax. Little did I know that down time would drive him even closer to his daemons."

"It was only later that I discovered it wasn't me or family that drove Todd to stay, the Admiral encouraged Todd to take a recently vacated position at NAVAIR, a Military Director of one of the largest competencies at the command."

The Admiral ordered Todd to take some leave before starting his next position, "I'm certain that if the Admiral didn't order him to take leave he wouldn't have." As it turns out Todd filled this time by taking multiple classes over the internet, painting the entire first two floors of the house, and of course exercising, often multiple times a day; "This was Todd's idea of relaxing."

After two weeks of leave Todd started his next job. Unaccustomed to the slower pace and having white space on his calendar he filled the voids with going to the gym and excising on the elliptical. "Todd would bring one set of clothes with him and tell me he worked out once a day. I knew it was more than that. He was working out more and more. On the weekends Todd would workout multiple times a day, sometime disappearing for multiple hours."

"Anything I asked Todd to do around the house he would do. He would just do it quickly, rushed, and not pay attention to any detail. He did it this way so that he could still work out."

"Todd was getting thinner. He had lost weight when he returned from Iraq and was now losing even more. At six feet tall he was down to about 140lbs. The muscular framed man I once knew was now a bunch of skin loosely hanging around his bones."

When I confronted Todd about his weight loss he simply deflected the conversation often just saying, "Don't worry about me. I'm fine." When I grew suspicious about how often he was working out during the day he would lie to me saying, "I just worked out twice." When in fact he worked out four or five times in a single day. "Todd was obsessed with working out."

"Unknown to me at the time, Todd had turned something that should have been considered 'healthy' into a form of self-harm. For Todd, exercising to extreme was a way to confront his daemons and if by doing so meant his early death, so be it."

Seurat Dot Thirty-Two
Kiss On The Dance Floor

Sharon and Todd's oldest son, Josh was engaged to be married. The wedding took place in mid-September, the first of their children to be married.

The morning of the rehearsal quickly approached. Sharon had taken the day off from her job at the High School. She awoke to Todd's vacated and cold sheets. Sharon headed down to the kitchen to discover that Todd had just finished his second one hour workout.

She asked Todd, "How many times have you worked out this morning?"

Todd replied, "Just a couple why?"

Sharon stated, "Don't you think that's obsessive?"

Todd became irritable. He knew she was right but he also knew that working out was his only way to make it through the day. "I'm not obsessing. I just like to work out. It's the one thing that makes me happy."

Sharon became visibly emotional. Her eyes welled up with tears, "I don't want to fight. Not today. Our son is getting married."

Todd responds, "I don't care. I'm tired of this."

Sharon looks at Todd, "What do you mean, THIS."

"THIS. I'm tired of it. I want out. I can't do this anymore."

Sharon responds, "So do you mean you don't want US anymore?"

Todd replies, "I want out of this. I just want this all to go away. I want a divorce." After saying these words, Todd reaches for his gym shoes and storms off to the basement to work out for yet a third time.

Sharon's in tears and emotionally upset over the discussion. She knows that she has to carry on with the mundane task that still needed to be done. She instinctively reaches for her keys, loads the trash into the back of the car, and heads toward the local dump. After throwing the trash into a bin at the dump Sharon pulls away and heads toward a nearby parking lot.

Sharon stops the car and tries to get her emotions under control. Holding back her tears she dials a friend from work on her cell phone. Sharon begins to explain all that has happened and asks for her advice and wisdom on how she should get through the next forty-eight hours. The discussion centered on the importance of their son and the importance of making everything appear as normal as possible. Sharon would need to address their marital issues once the wedding was over.

Todd finished his third workout, showered in the basement, and headed back up the stairs. Sharon, now home, was still visibly upset, "Can we just make it through this weekend. You owe that much to Josh. We need to try and not ruin Josh's day."

Todd, physically and emotionally exhausted agreed, "Yea. I'll be fine."

Few words were shared between the two of them as they packed the car and headed toward the hotel where the reception was to be held.

They arrived at the hotel in time to check-in and place their bags in the room before having to head to the church for the rehearsal. Before Sharon and Todd left the hotel for the church Todd headed down the stairs to the gym, elated to see multiple elliptical machines. Unbeknownst to Sharon, Todd had already made a mental plan, "Just get through the rehearsal, the dinner, and get back to the hotel. Then I'll workout."

Following the rehearsal the wedding party went to a nearby restaurant for the traditional rehearsal dinner. Sharon and Todd made it through the dinner although Sharon could tell that Todd was not happy. Soon after they arrived in the room Sharon went to go visit with family who flew in for the wedding. Todd excused himself, headed back to the room, changed into shorts and a T-Shirt, and headed to the hotel gym. He worked out that night for nearly two hours. When he got back to the room he said very little to Sharon. He showered and simply went to bed.

The morning of the wedding was filled with the usual preparations. Todd woke around 5:00 in the morning, headed to the gym, and worked out for an hour and a half before returning to shower and change into his uniform.

Sharon and Todd arrived at the church about an hour early for photos and pre wedding preparations. After the wedding and on the way to the reception Todd grasped Sharon's hand saying, "I'm sorry. I don't want us to be done with. I don't want a divorce. I know something is wrong. I know I need to get help. Monday I will call the flight doc. I'll get back on the meds and start seeing the therapist again. We're more important than the flight pay and my flight status. I finally realize that now."

Sharon had her doubts and reservations. She thought to herself….. "Maybe this is our rock bottom. Maybe we can go up from here."

Ironically one of the photos' taken at the reception is one of Sharon and Todd locked in kiss as they danced on the floor at their son's wedding reception. Just behind them, in the frame, stand their son Josh and his new bride. This photo now sits in their family room, right beneath the television and in clear sight. For Sharon, the picture represents a new beginning. A second chance and even HOPE.

The day was not just the start of their son's wedding vows but the reaffirmation of their own love for one another. A love that has lasted, stood the test of time, weathered the storm of sickness and despair, and frequent separations.

That December, Sharon and Todd celebrated their 25th Wedding anniversary. They held a surprise anniversary party in their Son and Daughter-in-Laws new home.

Sharon had always loved one particular black and white photo Todd had taken of the three children in Monterey. The picture shows Josh, Zach, and Rebekah all in various poses on stumps located in the backyard of their military housing. It was Sharon's favorite.

Todd had the picture enlarged and placed on a canvas. Unbeknownst to Sharon, he had coordinated with his daughter-in-law to have it shipped, wrapped, and waiting at their house. During the surprise anniversary party, Todd presented the picture to Sharon.

At the moment Sharon opened the gift and got the first sight of what was inside, Sharon threw her arms up in the air and out to her sides while screaming happily. The picture of that moment remains one of Todd's favorite. The picture captures the pure joy that his wife brings to each day, an enduring, and persistent love.

Section Five
A Spouses S.E.A.M.

This book highlighted for me, and hopefully others, depression IS NOT *singular* in its effect. My wife and I demonstrated this fact though some thirty-two *Seurat Experience Dots*. The following pages will expand on the S.E.A.M. process describing how the steps were applied.

A Spouse's Seurat Experience Dot Revealed

The Seurat Experience Dots outlined in the previous pages highlight the first portion of the SEAM process. The dots portrayed a review of my wife's life experiences. Arguably, not a complete list, they do however, represent some of the most influential. The following is provided as an outline only. Each step is provided a reference back to the original process step described in detail within the *Mending the S.E.A.M.: A Process for Enhancing Traditional Depression Therapies.*

The Experience List (Ref Page 32)

My wife and I combed through her list of experiences, culling through the subjects to pick out those specific dots we felt played a role in my depression OR, Sharon's ability to coop with it. Figure 1, *Experience List (Example)*, represents just one of the six pages Sharon generated.

The process was often times difficult to get through. The empty wad of Kleenex lying in the garbage a testament to the tearful memories and anguish surrounding these seemingly unrelated events.

The Chronological List (Ref Page 36)

The second step involved sorting Sharon's original list and ordering the happenings from earliest to latest occurrence. Figure 2, *Chronologic List (Example)* is a graphic representation of just one page in her chronologically sorted list.

The Experience Decomposition (Ref Pages 47 - 55)

Figure 3 depicts the result of the decomposition process of various influence factors such as Duration (or dwell), Emotion, Physical Environment, and People. Sharon used the emotions listed on page 42 of the *S.E.AM.* and simply associated them with her unique experience. A similar approach was conducted when evaluating both environment factors.

Self-Analysis Matrix (Ref Pages 56-70)

After Sharon completed decomposing each experience we began to look at what the information was telling us. We developed some simple matrix diagrams presented as Figures 4 through 6.

A Complete SEURAT Experience Dot

After complete the basic task described we associated one of three sized circles (Large, Medium, and Small), filling in the circle with a color of either white, grey, or black. The completed *Seurat Experience Dot* is placed at the beginning of each unique experience. Developed to represent a visual presentation of the writing.

The diameter of the dot represented the contribution of factors described in the second book. These factors were each considered and assigned a value that when summed, equated to one of the three sized circles.

The smaller more constrained circle represented a significant contribution by all the factors, assuming each factor is equally weighted. The larger circles, represented a less constrained or less contribution of the factors.

The Seurat Experience Dots themselves were colored using a standard grey scale pallet. Unlike Seurat, who utilized multiple colors to create beautiful images and scenes, I simply decided to use white, grey, and black.

The color white equated to an emotion or set of emotions that ranked higher on the scale described in the SEAM book. Emotions that tended to lie in the area of being good or happy.

Grey equated to a range of emotions. Typically and simply stated, a grey color was assigned when emotions ranged from happy to sad.

Black was assigned when the predominate mood or emotion set were grouped toward emotions typically associated with a death in the family or dying.

Using the above process I could depict an overall sense of the experience utilizing a simple dot, filled with either white, grey or black coloring.

The beginning of each of the four sections presented a collage of dots. The college of Seurat Experience Dots were taken from the pages that preceded each section. They were grouped randomly by me in attempt to portray an image of life experiences.

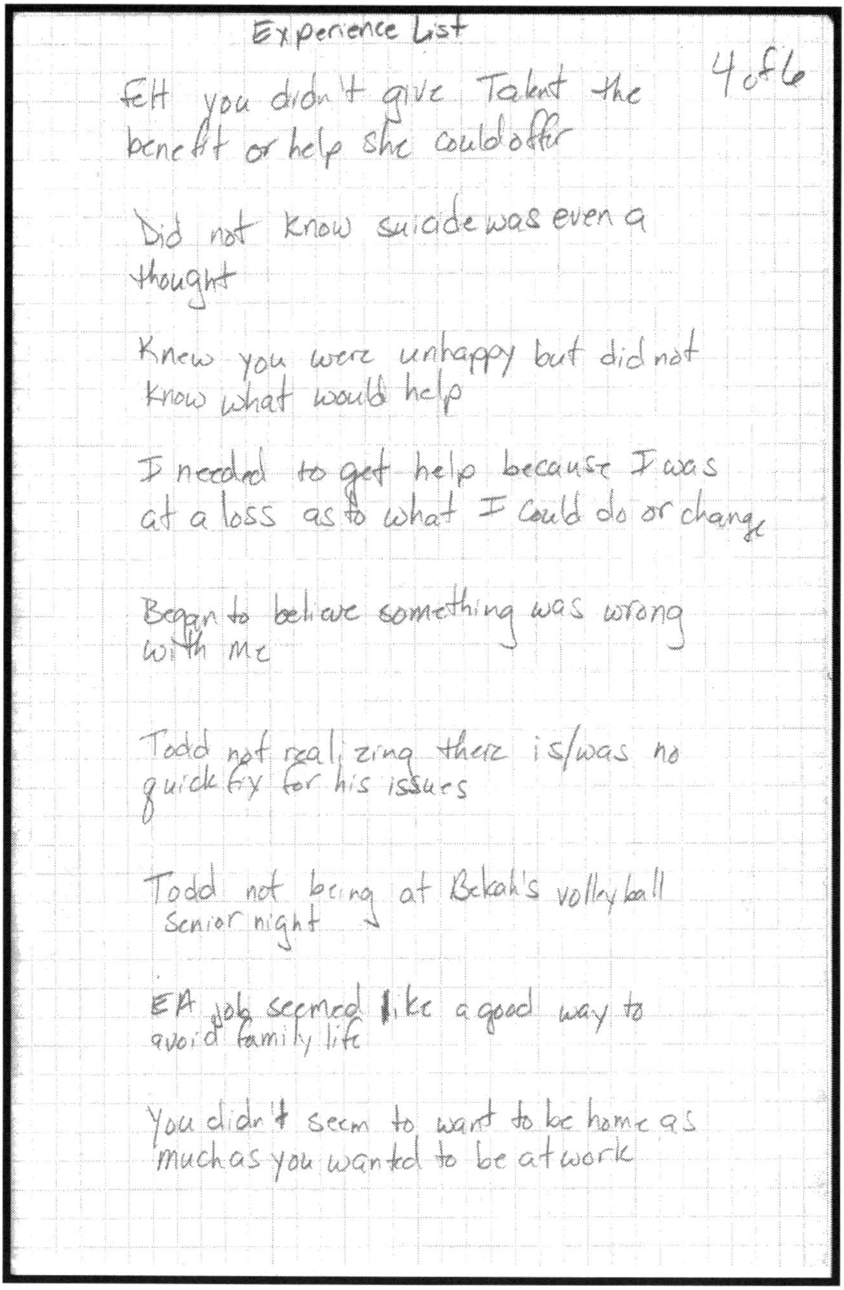

Experience List

4 of 6

Felt you didn't give Talent the benefit or help she could offer

Did not know suicide was even a thought

Knew you were unhappy but did not know what would help

I needed to get help because I was at a loss as to what I could do or change

Began to believe something was wrong with me

Todd not realizing there is/was no quick fix for his issues

Todd not being at Bekah's volleyball senior night

EA job seemed like a good way to avoid family life

You didn't seem to want to be home as much as you wanted to be at work

Figure 1. Experience List (example)

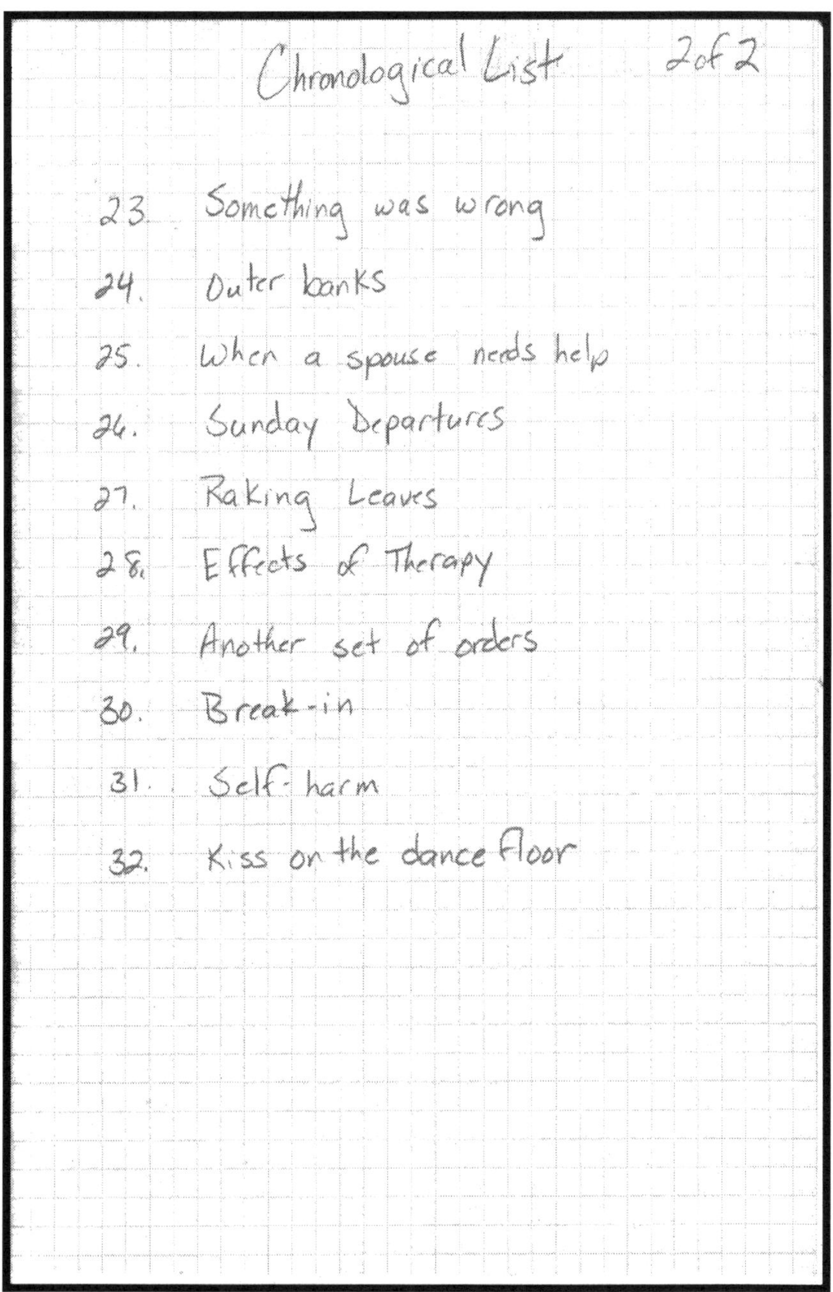

Figure 2. Chronological Experience List (example)

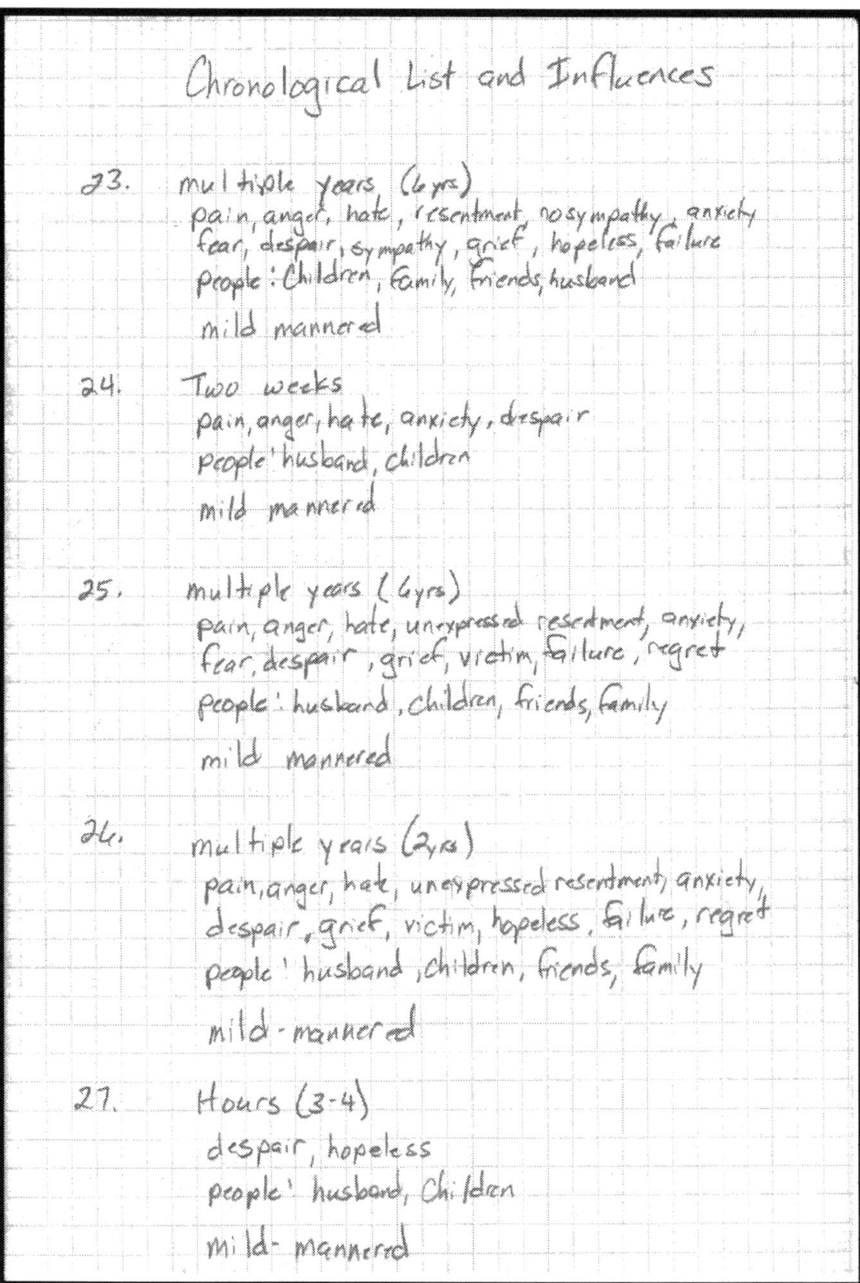

Chronological List and Influences

23. multiple years (6 yrs)
pain, anger, hate, resentment, no sympathy, anxiety
fear, despair, sympathy, grief, hopeless, failure
people: Children, family, friends, husband
mild mannered

24. Two weeks
pain, anger, hate, anxiety, despair
people: husband, children
mild mannered

25. multiple years (6 yrs)
pain, anger, hate, unexpressed resentment, anxiety,
fear, despair, grief, victim, failure, regret
people: husband, children, friends, family
mild mannered

26. multiple yrars (2 yrs)
pain, anger, hate, unexpressed resentment, anxiety,
despair, grief, victim, hopeless, failure, regret
people: husband, children, friends, family
mild-mannered

27. Hours (3-4)
despair, hopeless
people: husband, Children
mild-mannered

Figure 3. Chronological List and Influences (example)

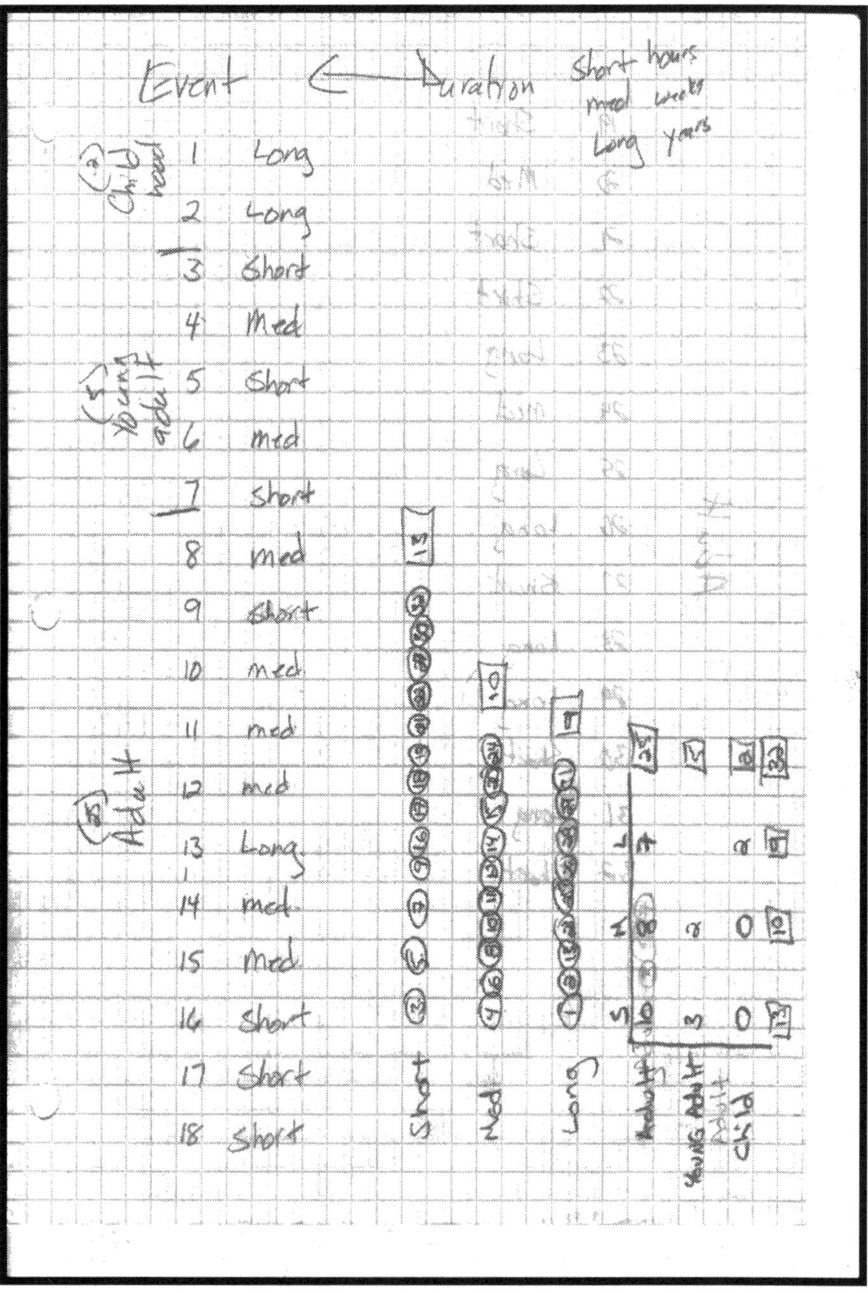

Figure 4. Influence Matrix (Duration)

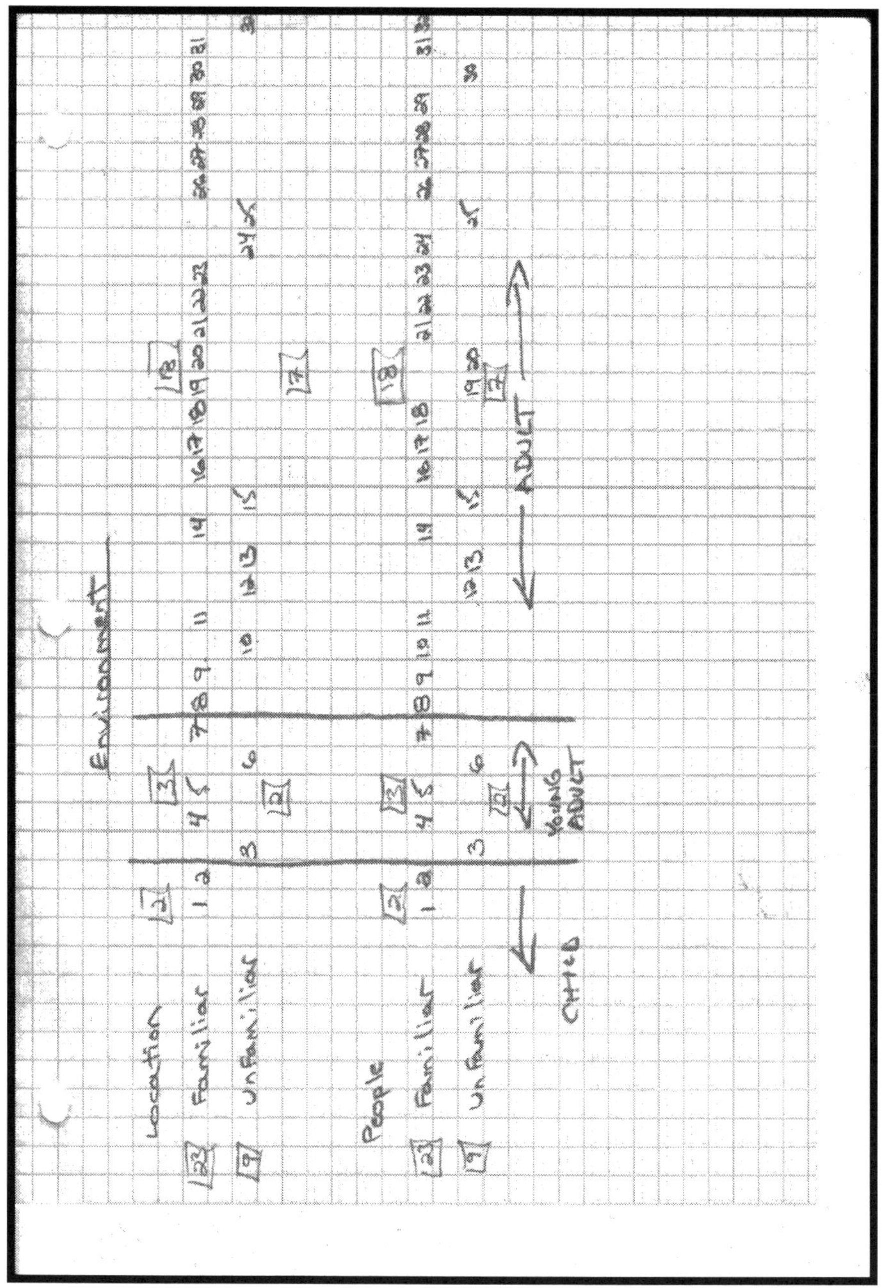

Figure 5. Influence Matrix (Environment and People)

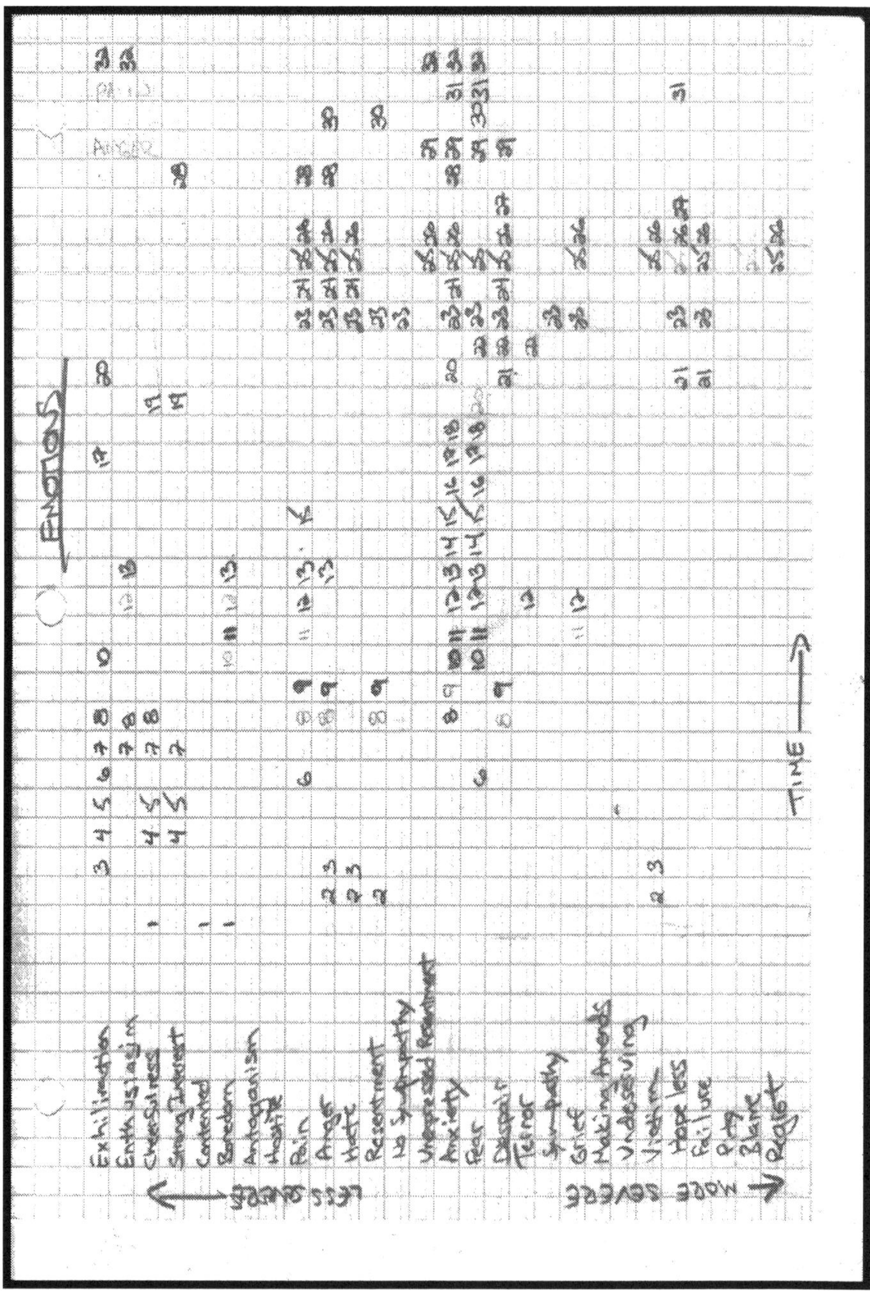

Figure 6. Emotions List

A Spouses Lucius Emotional Vein Revealed (Ref pages 81-88)

The S.E.A.M process culminates in depicting each dot as a three dimensional piece of a *Lucius Emotional Vine.* An attempt has been made to represent these individual segments in Figure 7. Once the individual segments are layered and or placed in parallel with one another, we begin to see a more complete representation. Figure 8, *My Spouses Lucius Emotional Vein Segment* is simply an example of what these seemingly disparate experiences look like when viewed as a whole.

Filling in the vein structure revealed to us several specifics of the past six years. The predominant emotions Sharon has been dealing with have been Anger, Hate, Anxiety, Fear, Despair, and Pain. In Sharon's case, emotions were the dominate trait when compared with other influences such as environment and duration.

The vein indicates a thickening or constriction beginning in 2008 and lasting for the most part until present day, 2014. The thickening or constraining aligns with Todd's return from his Iraq deployment.

Although the process was difficult, at times emotionally draining, Todd pointed out to Sharon something he saw in the analysis, "We're getting better." Todd was quick to point out Sharon's choice of emotions related to the last Seurat Experience Dot. It's often said that one data point does not represent a trend. Todd would agree. However, the dot does represent HOPE to the two of them. HOPE that Todd's continued treatment coupled with Sharon's support and understanding will give them a future. Another twenty-five years of marriage. Twenty-five years more time to create even more DOTS. Time to extend the length of their emotional vein and HOPE for better days to come.

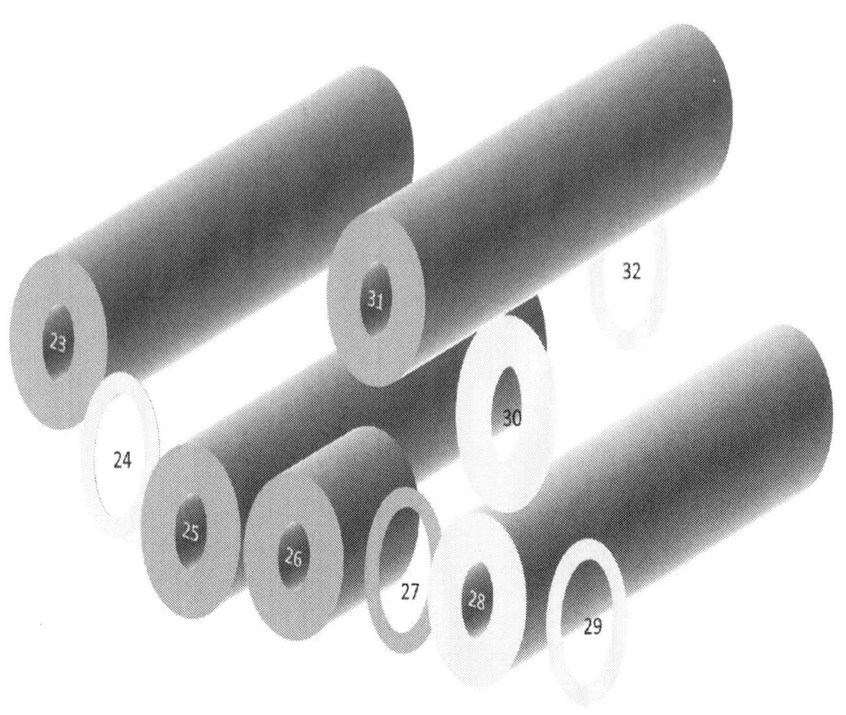

Figure 7. Lucius Emotional Vein Segments

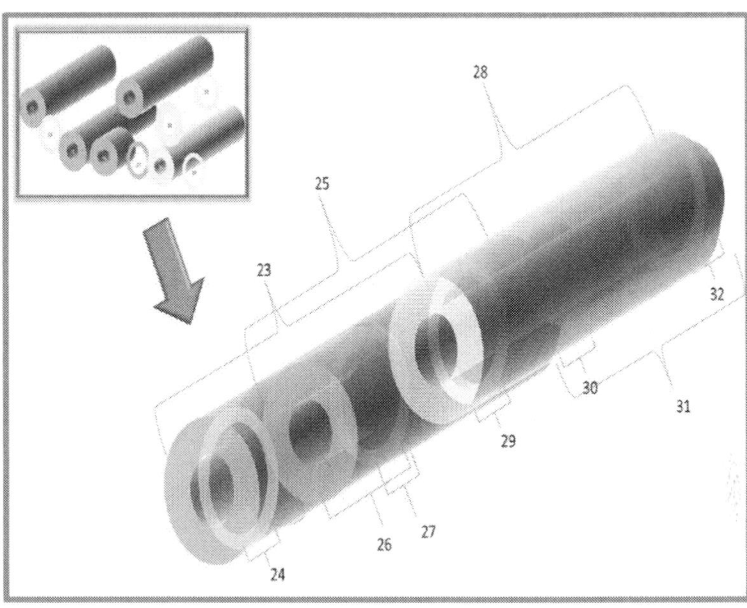

Figure 8. My Spouses Lucius Emotional Vein (segment)

Epilogue

By Sharon Kruder

I was very optimistic when Todd first decided to go for therapy. I thought things were heading in the right direction – the right path. Todd seemed to think medication alone was the answer, he went to talk therapy but he went reluctantly which I feel decreased its value.

Once Todd found out what effect being on a medication or in a therapy for depression longer than six months would have on his flight pay and fight status he stopped his medication and left therapy. I tried to explain to Todd his health and wellbeing were more important than money. Todd didn't share this belief with me. Being the bread winner in the household was his top priority. Seeing his paycheck decremented over an illness he had little or no control over was more than he wanted to bear. He basically chose money and career over family.

When Todd was in therapy, I could see the old Todd coming back. But when he was out of therapy he was miserable to be around.

The stigma surrounding depression and mental health is real. It wasn't until Todd finally was able to rationalize the stigma, he stuck to a treatment plan. Although, in some way, I think Todd had a right to be disappointed. He served his time; he met all the flight gates, and he was in better shape physically than most his age. How could I explain this outcome?

Due to this stigma, Todd removed himself from therapy twice before he realized the damage and hurt he imparted on his family. **You, the spouse, maybe the only thing that can lead them to help.**

Depression is conniving, it lies, it deceives, and it can kill. Your spouse who suffers from depression must want help. **Guide them toward this choice.** The decision to get help must come from the person needing help. **You just need to keep providing them encouragement to make that choice.**

In many ways Todd is still obsessed. Or, maybe, just maybe, terrified of what he may become if he should stop or slow down. Will he revert back to the loneliness, the isolation, and dark thoughts of his depression? Will he consider suicide once again as the answer to his problems? Will he find that the last chapter, the last sentence, the last word, and the last period he types be the moment he decides to leave this world?"

By not giving up, being relentless, we will face this depression together and become more resilient than ever before….. This **IS** my hope.

In Todd's first book he used the term "ships bell" as a metaphor for those offering help and assistance. As a military spouse I think the "ships bell" can best be described as **OUR RELENTLESSNESS, OUR PASSION, and**

OUR LOVE we give to our military members, veterans and their families. **So ring the bell, ring it loudly, and ring it often.**

As I write this, Todd and I are still on this *Journey in the Fog of Depression.* We keep on finding ways to deal with depression in our lives. **Our experience with depression is not over. It is still going on. BE RELENTLESS and DON'T GIVE UP! Remember, there IS always HELP and there IS always HOPE.**

End Note

On behalf of the authors and their entire family, we thank you for taking the time to read about our experiences. We hope the material contained within these pages will provide you hope. Hope that your illness can be managed and hope that you will find your way through the darkness of the fog.

This is the third of four planned writing on the subject of depression by the same author and released in partnership with Seurat Innovations, LLC, and a social enterprise company.

Together, these books will be a compendium of knowledge the author openly intends to share to benefit others suffering day-day with the illness of depression.

A portion of the proceeds from the sale of these titles will go directly to further the Lucius Seneca Wellness Group Inc. A Maryland Non-Profit and companion company of Seurat Innovations, LLC.

Lucius Seneca Wellness Group will distribute, at no cost, paper copies of the titles, making them freely available to military Behavioral Health Centers and Family Support Centers.

The two companies, Seurat Innovations and Lucius Seneca Wellness Group share in the ideals of improving the behavioral health of our military, veterans, and their families.

More information about these two companies can be found on their websites; www.SeuratInnovations.com and www.LuciusSenecaWG.org.

"The only journey is the one within."
— Rainer Maria Rilke

About the Authors

Captain and Mrs. Todd Kruder have been married for over twenty-five years. Captain Kruder has accumulated over twenty-five years of faithful and dedicated service to our Nation as a military officer while Sharon shared in his dedicated service raising five children while dutifully accompanying him on numerous permanent change of station orders. In the fall of 2008, Captain Kruder was diagnosed with severe depression. The couple hopes that by sharing their story, others will find help and hope in their own journey with depression.

Synopsis

The *Journey in the Fog of Depression: A Military Spouse's Experience* is a unique view into the life of a Military Spouse and her personal accounting of the events and effects of her husband's depression.

Written in a narrative style, the authors describe in detail, the events, challenges, and experiences of what life is like married to a military officer. We learn how the early challenges of their marriage and the frequent deployments instilled in her, the strength and determination to save the life of her spouse.

A compelling description of relentless perseverance and hope.

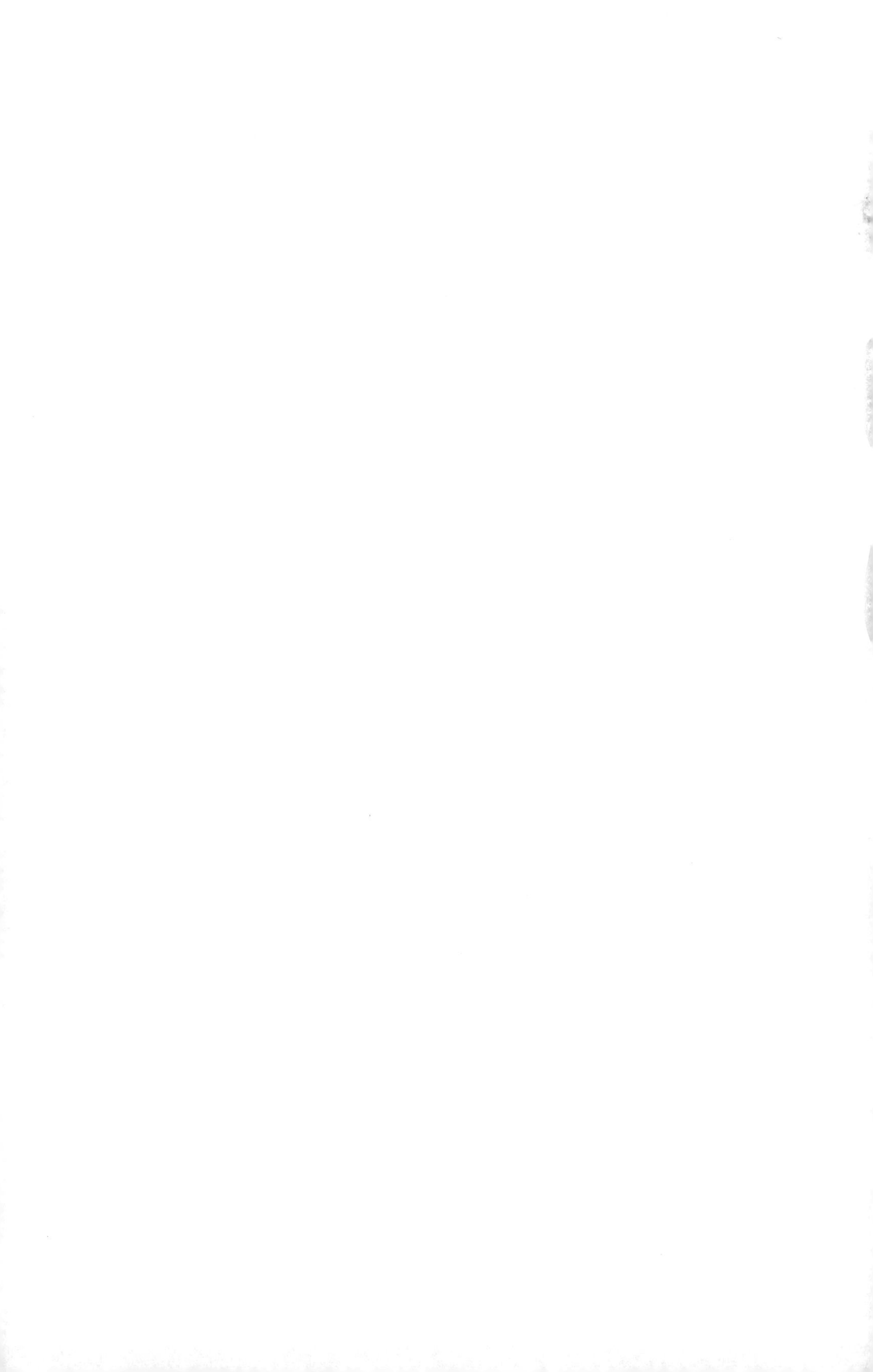

Proof

Made in the USA
Charleston, SC
31 March 2014